Advance Praise for *Stand by Her:*

"In the din of self-help books and personal memoirs, *Stand by Her* distinguishes itself as a welcome and steady voice of wisdom. John Anderson skillfully describes the emotional impact a cancer diagnosis can have on family members and caregivers as they try to make sense of a profoundly chaotic and devastating experience. *Stand by Her* suggests ways for men to stay connected with the emotional aspects of the experience without getting lost in the details of the 'business of cancer.' It represents a unique contribution and is a valuable resource."

> —Penny Damaskos, LCSW, OSW-C, Coordinator of the
> Post-Treatment Resource Program, Memorial
> Sloan-Kettering Cancer Center

"John Anderson takes the reader through the terrifying, frustrating, and unfamiliar world of a woman's breast cancer diagnosis with humor, frankness, and practical advice gleaned from experts and a lot of personal experience. Anyone supporting a loved one with any kind of cancer will benefit from this book, but it should be required reading for the men in the life of a breast cancer patient, whether they be husbands, fathers, brothers, ex-spouses, sons, or close friends."

> —Hala Moddelmog, President and CEO, Susan G. Komen
> for the Cure®

"This book is an amazing resource. Informative, funny, moving, and always brutally frank, it is a must for men (and women!) trying to understand the world of breast cancer."

> —Barron H. Lerner, MD, Professor of Medicine, Columbia
> University, and author, *The Breast Cancer Wars*

"*Stand by Her* is an accurate and heartfelt description of the emotions and feelings a spouse goes through during discovery and treatment of breast cancer. If you have already gone through the process, it makes you feel like you're not alone. If you are about to, it will give you an excellent understanding of what to expect."

> —Frank Fiorina, husband of cancer survivor Carly Fiorina,
> ex-CEO, Hewlett-Packard

Stand by Her

A Breast Cancer Guide for Men

....

John W. Anderson

⁞AMACOM

AMERICAN MANAGEMENT ASSOCIATION

New York • Atlanta • Brussels • Chicago • Mexico City • San Francisco
Shanghai • Tokyo • Toronto • Washington, D.C.

This publication is designed to provide accurate and authoritative information in regard to the subject
matter covered. It is sold with the understanding that the publisher is not engaged in rendering legal,
accounting, or other professional service. If legal advice or other expert assistance is required, the services
of a competent professional person should be sought.

The ideas, procedures, and suggestions contained in this book are not intended as a substitute for
consulting your healthcare provider. All matters regarding the health of the breast cancer patient
require medical supervision. Neither the publisher nor the author shall be liable or responsible for any
loss or damage allegedly arising from any information or suggestions in this book.

Quote from "Refugee" on page 150 is copyright © Tom Petty and Michael Campbell, Tarka Music,
adm. by Almo Music Corp. (ASCAP). Used by permission. Quote from "Don't Do Me Like That"
on page 150 is copyright © Tom Petty, Tarka Music, adm. by Almo Music Corp. (ASCAP). Used
by permission.

Library of Congress Cataloging-in-Publication Data

Anderson, John W., 1959–
    Stand by her : a breast cancer guide for men / John W. Anderson.
        p.   cm.
    Includes index.
    ISBN-13: 978-0-8144-1391-3 (pbk.)
    ISBN-10: 0-8144-1391-9 (pbk.)
    1. Breast—Cancer—Patients—Family relationships. 2. Husbands. I. Title.
    RC280.B8A4945 2010
    616.99'449—dc22

                                                                            2009015461

Printing number

10   9   8   7   6   5   4   3

CONTENTS

·················· F O R E W O R D ······················

In my practice, I treat women with every stage of breast cancer and those who are at high risk for developing breast cancer. I see women who are in their twenties and in their nineties, who work, who care for their children or their elderly parents, who live alone, who are married, single, widowed, divorced, straight, gay, who come from every corner of New York City and its environs. For each of these women and those who love her, the breast cancer journey is unique. Nonetheless there are similarities and shared experiences in the process of diagnosis and treatment. John Anderson knows this. He lived through breast cancer with his mother and then his wife was diagnosed. His sister and a dear family friend were also affected. John faced this ordeal too many times, and each time he was there for his loved one.

Although most women in America do not die of breast cancer, many fear breast cancer more than any other illness. In the last decades, this fear has motivated women to speak out and demand that attention be paid. Because of breast cancer advocacy groups, the women's movement, committed physicians, and scientists who do innovative laboratory work and carefully conducted clinical research, we continue to change the standards of practice. We have made great progress in both the science and the art of treating this complex spectrum of diseases that we call breast cancer.

Still, more than 150,000 women will be diagnosed with breast cancer in America each year. They will face difficult decisions about surgery and systemic therapy, chemotherapy, radiation, hormonal therapy, and biologic treatment. Treatment will impact their bodies and their minds, their hearts and their spirits. Research data confirm the notion that emotional and psychosocial support for breast cancer patients is beneficial in many ways.[1] A wealth of resources, information, and support services are available for breast cancer patients. But for their loved ones? Not nearly enough.

What about the men who love these women? Most are completely unprepared for the trauma of learning that a woman he is close to has been diagnosed with breast cancer. Then figuring out his role and how to be present and loving and helpful—while maintaining a sense of himself—is daunting. John lived through breast cancer first as a son, then a young husband, a brother, and a dear friend. He has truly stood by the women he loves who have been affected by breast cancer. And, in each instance, he found what was shared and what was special. In each instance, he did figure out how to be with her, to support her, to help navigate the medical world, to listen, take notes, tell jokes, give hugs, work, carpool, organize, cook, watch movies, and hold her in his arms. *Stand by Her* is as much personal memoir as it is guide for the perplexed. With just the right touch of humor and practicality, John takes on what terrifies us the most.

We will continue to work in the laboratory and in the clinic to understand the biology of breast cancer—to develop more effective targeted therapies, with less toxicity and better quality of life. We will continue to work together, doctors and patients, in shared decision making, in clinical trials research, studying epidemiology and genetics, to treat and to prevent breast cancer. As we move forward in this effort, we must also carry with us the emotional and psychological toll that breast cancer takes not only on the woman who is diagnosed, but on everyone in her sphere. We must now pay attention to these men and women as well.

Stand by Her is the best beginning for men traveling the breast cancer journey with the women they love.

Ruth Oratz, MD, FACP
Clinical Associate Professor of Medicine
New York University School of Medicine
Founder and Director
The Women's Oncology & Wellness Practice, New York City

Note

1. Candyce H. Kroenke, Laura D. Kubzansky, Eva S. Schernhammer, Michelle D. Holmes, and Ichiro Kawachi, "Social Networks, Social Support, and Survival After Breast Cancer Diagnosis," *Journal of Clinical Oncology* 24, no. 7 (March 1, 2006): 1105–1111.

To Sharon:

Breast Cancer Survivor, Advocate
Wife
Mother
Business Partner
Best Friend
Soul Mate

·············· A C K N O W L E D G M E N T S ···············

This book began when my mom, Anne Anderson, was first diagnosed with breast cancer back in January 1978, and took twenty-one years to complete—during which time my wife, Sharon Rapoport, my sister, Mary Enright, and my mom's best friend, Caryl Spease, were diagnosed too. But it was the selfless support and commitment to this project of my wife Sharon that made this book possible. It was Sharon who carried the major workload of our company, The Farm, to give me time to write. She deserves the greatest thanks of all, for without her, this book would never have been written, let alone published. Sharon, I love you so much, more than I could ever express in words here, as my wife, best friend, and business partner. Mary, Caryl, and of course Mom, thanks so much for inspiring me to finish this as well.

I want to thank my dear sweet dad, William P. Anderson Jr., for being such an inspiration to me, not only as a loving father but also as the very first caregiver whom I saw giving so much love to my mom each and every day throughout her ten-year battle with breast cancer. When I was born, my dad wanted to name me William Pennell Anderson III—nickname Penn—which would have been a perfect name for a writer. My mom, however, would have nothing to do with that. But she did concede William as my middle name, and so Dad, I want to say how proud I am to have your name, given all that you have shown me by example of being not only a good man, but a great one.

Then there is my other dad, my father-in-law Dr. Jack Rapoport, who stood by his daughter, and me, every step of the way as we all traveled together through Cancer Land. If there's a more dedicated father to his daughter than Jack Rapoport, I want to meet him.

I want to thank my two sons, Seth and Isaac. They were just 7 and 5 when their mom was first diagnosed. Seth and Isaac stood by her every step of the way, from hugging her right after surgery in her hospital room to making her laugh after a tough chemo treatment to now marching by her side at Race for the Cure events as teenage boys taller than she is, standing proud alongside her for her accomplishments as a breast cancer survivor and as an incredible advocate for Susan G. Komen For the Cure.

There are my brothers to thank—Steve, Mike, Terry, and Chris; and Bubba (aka Kevin), the youngest, who stood right beside me to console me right after I had just found out that Sharon had been diagnosed. Bubba never left my side, or Sharon's, until she was fully recovered after her final treatment.

Sarah Hazlegrove, when you stepped into our house to do the heavy lifting of all the thankless cooking, cleaning, and scrubbing around the house, while at the same time arbitrating all the emotional struggles between a harried husband, wife, and children, you became a Mother Teresa meets Mrs. Clean superhero. Mary Rapoport, thank you so much for running our home better than the Four Seasons when Sharon and I didn't know which way was up through her treatment. I want to also thank Mary Anderson, my dad's wife and my beloved stepmom, for being there for him as he struggled while his daughter and his daughter-in-law went through breast cancer at the same time.

I can't forget my Bromancers—André Bernard and Bill Oberlander especially, Guy Lawson and Paul Blum, and my Bromancerettes—Jenny Bernard, Susan Brecker, Dale Oberlander, and Jane Waldrop—who got me through the toughest of times.

Then there are the doctors, who are the true force behind stopping breast cancer for life. I want to especially thank Dr. Bonnie

Reichman for checking, and correcting, all the medical information in this book. I also want to send out a special thanks to Dr. Barron Lerner, who was not only an incredible medical advocate for my wife's treatment, but also became a great friend to her and to me. Thanks to Dr. Ruth Oratz, Dr. Beth Ann Ditkoff, Dr. Randy Stevens, Dr. Jeffrey Ascherman, and Dr. Suzen Merten for all their help. Thanks are in high order to Lisa Baroni and Penny Damaskos for helping my family navigate all the emotional and psychological tsunamis thrown our way by breast cancer.

This book is in your hands because of my agent, Jane Dystel, who believed in this project from the moment I told her about it on the phone. Jane, you're the greatest. Thanks to Miriam Goderich, Jane's business partner at Dystel & Goderich, for all your help too. Kelly O'Dell Stanley, I really appreciate all of your creative input. And a big thanks goes out for the valuable work put into this book by all my editors at AMACOM—Stan Wakefield, Barry Richardson, and Erika Spelman.

Special thanks goes out to Jay Foster and his wife Brenda, who agreed to use this book before it was even finished while Brenda was going through treatment. The way you two handled your journey is an inspiration to us all.

I will never forget, or ever be able to properly thank, all the men and women who bravely shared with me the personal stories about breast cancer that are contained here. It is my hope that these stories will help the millions more following in their footsteps.

Finally I want to thank Lydia Oswald, who is, I believe, the most elegant woman to have ever walked on the face of this Earth. Lydia, a breast cancer *and* Holocaust survivor, believed in this book's mission—to help men when their loved ones are diagnosed—as much as or more than anyone else. She beat Nazi Germany, she beat breast cancer, but unfortunately she couldn't beat ovarian cancer, dying with incredible dignity last year at the age of 93. But her spirit lives on, I hope, within the pages of this book.

INTRODUCTION

．．．．．．．．．．．．．．．．．．．．．．

SOMEONE VERY CLOSE TO you, right now, is either under-going treatment for breast cancer or has just been diagnosed. It could be your wife, your mother, your sister, your daughter, your girlfriend, your grandmother, your aunt, your cousin, your friend, or your office mate. No matter who she is, she needs *you*. That's why you're holding this book in your hands.

Every three minutes, a woman in the United States is told she has breast cancer—over 184,000 in 2008. That translates to one in every eight American women. Worldwide, approximately 1.2 million cases of breast cancer were diagnosed in 2008, according to the World Health Organization. There are currently over two million breast cancer survivors living in the United States.

The Journal of Oncology Practice reported that cancer diagnoses will increase significantly over the next twenty years, owing to the ever-growing population of Americans sixty-five years and older, a number expected to double between 2000 and 2030. The American Society of Clinical Oncology has expressed concern that there is a critical shortage of oncologists, despite the fact that there are over 25,000 practicing members today. The National Cancer Institute (NCI) plans to add fifteen more cancer centers across the country over the next five years to bolster the sixty already in existence. The NCI budget topped $5 billion.

For these reasons, and many more like them, *Dr. Susan Love's Breast Book: 4th Edition,* by Susan Love (Da Capo Press, 2005) is

3

the Amazon.com number-two best-seller on the subject of women's health. Yet there is not one comprehensive guidebook available today that talks directly to men on what to do when the women in their lives get breast cancer—until now, with *Stand by Her*.

This book is written for men who want to be there for their loved ones when they are diagnosed with breast cancer. *Stand by Her* provides strategies and guidance on the countless medical and emotional minefields men face, every day, as husbands, fathers, sons, brothers, cousins, friends, and coworkers of breast cancer patients. Each chapter is a stage in the process, with its own unique color that symbolizes the feelings you are having and will face.

Combining personal anecdotes (I have stood by four women who went through this experience: my wife, my sister, my mom, and my mom's best friend) and the experiences of others, with information from professionals in medical, psychological, family relationship, sexual, and financial areas, *Stand by Her* is a step-by-step program targeted to men who want to become invaluable caregivers for their loved ones with breast cancer, while also helping men address and overcome their personal fears, frustrations, and anxieties that are caused by this disease. (All names other than the ones of those who are part of my personal story have been changed to protect the privacy of the patients and their loved ones.)

This book is just the beginning for caregivers, for there's also an accompanying website, www.standbyher.org, where readers can share their experiences anonymously. *Stand by Her* is also for breast cancer patients, for it offers women insights into the difficulties and challenges that their caregivers will face during the course of this disease; and it's also helpful for breast surgeons, oncologists, radiologists, nurses, and others among the support staff who treat patients with this disease every day. Indeed, discussions are currently under way with doctors and hospitals across the country to find ways to integrate *Stand by Her* methods into the breast cancer treatment system, so as to make caregivers a greater part of the treatment process.

Chances are, you've just received the bad news. And you've got a problem, a *big* problem: you have no idea what to do next. You are about to be initiated into an exclusive men's club, a group millions strong of men who have traveled the difficult journey you are about to undertake. Welcome to the *Stand by Her* brotherhood. We begin with the first step: diagnosis.

CHAPTER 1

The Abyss

"I Have Breast Cancer"

· ·

YOU'RE NEVER READY when "it" happens.

"I have breast cancer."

"It's malignant."

"They want to take my breasts."

"I need chemo."

"I have to get radiation."

Your world has just gone black. She's been diagnosed with breast cancer and you've just been dropped into a bottomless abyss.

· · ·

Sharon had it all. She was a successful creative director at a boutique advertising agency located in the hip SoHo section of New York City. Her client list included Coca-Cola, Colgate, CBS, the New York Yankees, MTV Networks, and *USA Today*. She was happily married to her business partner, with a nice house in Westchester County, New York, which was constantly consumed by laughter from her two young boys, Seth and Isaac, ages 7 and 5.

She was very excited about her latest client conquest, Lifetime Television. Sharon had been put in charge of creating a breast cancer public service campaign for the cable TV network, designed to encourage women to get yearly checkups from their doctors, have mammograms, and do monthly self-exams. Sharon learned during the creative briefing that one in eight women in the United States is diagnosed with breast cancer every year. The statistic made her stop and think: which of her friends would be the unlucky one?

At forty-one, Sharon had never had a mammogram. Women are encouraged to have their first breast screening by age 40, with some studies recommending as young as 35. Not to worry, Sharon thought. No one in my family has ever had breast cancer. Then she read that 85 percent of women who get breast cancer have no family history of it—just like her. Sharon crammed in a mammogram appointment to be just before she picked up her oldest child from elementary school. The actual visit was painless (other than the way they squished her breasts onto the machine, which hurt—a lot, actually). So, another to-do item had been crossed off her busy list. The phone rang several days later. The mammogram center name and number popped up on Sharon's caller ID: "We found an abnormality."

Abnormalities, it turns out, aren't that abnormal. Plenty of women are "diagnosed" every day with innocent, benign cysts in their breasts. That's what the mammogram center told her, before they recommended a breast surgeon in New York City who could take a biopsy of her suspicious lump. The first biopsy procedure Sharon had—fine needle aspiration, or FNA, as the docs like to call it—is quite simple: numb the area around the concerned spot, insert a very small needle, extract some cells, and test the suspected cells to see if they are cancerous. The surgeon decided to go one step further and do a core biopsy, which is similar to the fine needle procedure but uses a larger needle. Her biopsy results came back several days later: both inconclusive.

So the surgeon ordered a surgical lumpectomy to completely remove what he believed to be just a benign cyst. A frozen section was taken while Sharon was under general anesthesia. Still, nothing to worry about, she thought. While getting dressed after the procedure, the medical staff told Sharon that the surgeon needed to speak with her. It was then that Sharon first began to wonder—what if. When she was called into her doctor's office, the surgeon was on the phone, chatting away about an upcoming medical seminar that he was heading to in Ecuador, where he would teach one day and then spend the rest of his time on pristine golf courses framed by the Andes Mountains.

Sharon sat and listened as the surgeon bantered on about his golf short game. It made her relax. If he's more concerned about his sand wedge than her lump, she thought, surely everything was fine—just as it always had been. But the longer the phone call lasted, the more annoyed Sharon got sitting there, waiting, alongside her husband. Sharon had to get back to work on that breast cancer campaign to help all those women who were fighting breast cancer. Mustering up her best glare face, the surgeon got the message and hung up the phone. He looked at Sharon, and only at Sharon. He didn't acknowledge her husband at all.

"It's malignant."

Sharon is my wife.

• • •

Anne worked as an emergency room nurse. Everything and anything having to do with trauma came right to her in the ER: motorcycle accidents, newborn babies, heart attacks, strokes, brain aneurysms— the works. She loved the excitement and challenges she faced at St. Joseph's Hospital in Parkersburg, West Virginia. Sure, emergencies were stressful, but what a rush, she thought. To calm down after each shift, Anne lit up a cigarette, and on more eventful days, two or three during her ride home from the hospital.

One day, Anne got a call from her next-door neighbor, Mrs. Johnson, who needed medical help with her ailing husband, Jim. Upon entering the house, Anne heard a dreadful rattling sound, followed by an endless barrage of coughing and hacking. When Anne walked into Jim's bedroom, she saw the tent—an oxygen tent—under which Jim's terrified eyes met hers. He was suffocating, thanks to an incurable bout of emphysema.

Anne helped Jim clear his lungs of phlegm, then upped the oxygen level in the tent. Upon returning to her house, Anne went straight for her cigarette carton, tossed it in the trash can, and then sought out each of her three young boys—hugging each of them so tightly they could barely breathe. She swore never to smoke again. The next day, she quit her job at the ER and decided that her job for the rest of her life was to be a great mom.

Ten years later, Anne gave birth to her seventh child—a boy. There was no more room in her tiny three-bedroom, split-level house to fit her five other sons, one daughter, and husband, Bill. So Anne and Bill built a brand-new house just outside of town in one of those new developments where her kids could run wild and free in hundreds of wooded acres in back of their house. Even though Anne no longer worked at the hospital, she found a lot of reasons to visit the ER regularly. There was always a child dropping out of a tree, being cut by a knife, getting pushed down the stairs, blowing up firecrackers in his hands, melting plastic army men with gasoline, or falling off a bike when the speedometer hit 40 mph and the handlebars couldn't hold the road any longer.

Anne loved her life despite the daily madness of raising seven children. After her husband landed a big promotion as plant manager for a large chemical company on the East Coast, she looked forward to their country club cocktails every weekend after a long week of child chaos. When her youngest trotted off to elementary school, Anne enjoyed the sudden quiet in her house. But it didn't last long. The house was too quiet. So Anne signed up to be a nurse at a preschool nursery. One day, while holding her hands above her head to adjust her crisp white nursing cap, Anne felt a hot flash streak across her chest. Opening her blouse, she saw a huge red blotch splattered across her left breast. When she touched it, her face blanched. She felt a lump, and it was big.

Anne called her best friend to be by her side when she went in for surgery to remove the lump. Anne signed some forms, one of which said that if the surgeon found a malignant tumor, her breast would be removed. This was what doctors did back in 1978, before mammograms, sonograms, MRIs, or CAT and PET scans existed. As Anne was being sedated, she said a prayer. A devout Catholic, she prayed to St. John Neumann, an American saint credited for starting the first Catholic parochial schools in the United States. Then she stopped, in midprayer, and laughed because she was praying to a celibate priest to protect her bosom.

When Anne awoke in the recovery room after her operation, the first face she saw was her friend's, spattered with tears. Her friend gently took Anne's hand and placed it on Anne's left breast. Anne felt nothing. Her breast was gone. Anne had breast cancer; her tumor was the size of a walnut. Anne's survival prognosis was dismal. Her doctors gave her six months to live, tops.

Anne was my mom.

· · ·

Mary loved to run through the woods. The best part about it was that she could get away from everything—and everyone—by running as fast as she could, up and down hills, through streams, around trees, over rocks, full out. She was one of the premier runners on an all-girl cross-country team in Wilmington, Delaware. The team was the best in the state, ever; for that matter, it was one of the best in the country, ever. Mary and her teammates won the state title every year, helping her school, Padua Academy, rack up eight straight girls cross-country state championships in a row. When it was time to graduate and go to college, Mary didn't know what exactly she wanted to do (other than run, of course).

Mary attended the University of Delaware in Newark, Delaware, where she first declared business as her major, followed by sociology, then physical education after that. College was fun—a lot of fun. Mary, like most college kids, wanted to enjoy every moment of campus life, which she did until the phone rang one day in her dorm room. It was Mary's mom. Mary dropped the phone when she heard her mom say that her breast cancer was back again, for the third time. Mary was very close to her mom, and nothing—not even college—was more important. So Mary packed up her things, hugged her friends, and headed home to help her mom fight for her life.

Mary dutifully went to all her mom's chemo sessions, and she drove her mom to Philadelphia three times a week where they prayed together in front of a saint's shrine, while also doing the laundry, cooking the meals, and packing lunches for her dad and younger siblings. Mary was going to do whatever it took to keep her mom alive; unfortunately, that wasn't enough. Mary held her mom's hand when she died in a hospital bed on a cold March morning.

All of Mary's cross-country teammates came to the funeral. It was standing room only. Ten priests led the service that day. The scale of the ceremony felt like the church was burying a bishop. Mary was fine throughout the whole service, until they played her mom's favorite hymn, "On Eagle's Wings." "And He will raise you, up on eagle's wings." That's it, Mary thought. It was a direct calling, from her mom to her, to become a nurse, just like her mom had been.

Mary changed schools and graduated two years later with a nursing degree. She went into home care nursing so that she could provide a more personal touch to sick people's needs. When she met her future husband, Joe, she decided to move to Minnesota where he worked for Mayo Clinic. There was just one big problem with Mayo for Mary—its location. Minnesota was just too cold. So Mary convinced her husband, a Minnesota native, to transfer to another Mayo Clinic site in sunny Scottsdale, Arizona, where they moved their growing family of two boys, with a third boy on the way. Mary had been getting annual mammograms before any of her girlfriends even knew what the word meant. Mary had been checked and prodded so many times by doctors looking for cancer inside her that she thought maybe God had finally answered her prayers that cancer would not be part of her personal life, ever again. Then one day her doctor walked into the examination room with a blank stare on his face. "I have cancer, don't I?" she said to her doctor. The doctor didn't respond. He didn't have to. She knew.

Mary is my sister.

• • •

Caryl was always the first in her family to do everything. She was the first to be born, the first to attend college, the first to graduate college, the first to get married, and the first to have a child. She was also the first of her friends to hear about the awful tragedy that happened on a foggy night in Huntington, West Virginia, in November, 1970, when a chartered plane crashed, killing the entire Marshall University football team—seventy-five in all. Caryl was attending Marshall then, and had friends on that flight who were now dead. Classes were cancelled that day, and Caryl went to the memorial service held at the school stadium.

Life for Caryl after that crash changed forever; it was just too darn short. So Caryl got busy. She graduated early, got married, got pregnant, and had a daughter. Caryl moved to rural Pennsylvania to slow life down by growing her own garden and giving birth to two more daughters. Caryl loved being in the country, away from everything. She learned how to can peaches and make strawberry and blackberry jam. Her husband, Jerry, was a hunter, so she bought a deep freeze where she kept the deer meat that he bagged during hunting season. There was plenty to do around her old farmhouse— paint a room, fix a leaky faucet, patch a hole in the wall. Country living was just great—until an emergency happens.

Early one morning, Caryl awoke in a panic: she couldn't breathe. Her husband had already left for work. Desperate, Caryl knocked over a glass, which woke up her oldest daughter Christie, who came to her aid. Caryl was rushed to the hospital. The doctors were perplexed about what caused Caryl to stop breathing. They never did find out. But during the battery of tests, the doctors found a lump in her breast. The first person she called for help was Anne.

Caryl was my mom's best friend.

• • •

Twenty years later, and several cancer recurrences after, Caryl traveled to New York City to appear in a TV breast cancer campaign for

Lifetime Television called "Stop Breast Cancer for Life," standing alongside my wife, Sharon, who was still undergoing chemotherapy. I directed the spots. Caryl and Sharon are still here today. So is my sister Mary. My mom unfortunately didn't make it; after ten years of battle, she died on March 14, 1988.

She's Got Cancer

Bad news, when it comes, is all about location—you never forget where you were when it arrived. My first "big one" was President John F. Kennedy's assassination on November 22, 1963. I was pedaling furiously on my tricycle, going faster and faster around our family room to see if I could handle centrifugal force like my hero, Astronaut John Glenn. Then, I saw Walter Cronkite remove his glasses and rub a tear from his eyes as his voice cracked. I froze, as did the rest of the nation.

When my dad told me about my mom's diagnosis, I was standing in a classroom hallway at the University of Delaware, taking a break from studying for a midterm human anatomy final. When my mom's friend Caryl was diagnosed, I heard it from my mom, again on the phone, in my small Texas apartment after just getting back from Real Property Law class at the University of Houston Law School. When my wife Sharon was told about her breast cancer, I was sitting right next to her, holding her hand, in a tiny breast surgeon's office in midtown Manhattan, New York, as the snow floated down outside on a cold March day. When my sister Mary was diagnosed, I was home in New York watching the kids, when my wife told me after getting off the phone with my sister.

News of your loved one's breast cancer diagnosis has the same emotional impact as death, according to Delthia Ricks, author of

Breast Cancer Basics. Dr. Beth Ann Ditkoff, my wife's breast surgeon at Columbia Presbyterian Hospital in New York City, says, "A breast cancer diagnosis is like a house on fire that is burning to the ground. It is an extraordinary diagnosis, and the worst thing of all is that the patient and their loved ones almost always have no experience about what to do about it."

Richard, of Kansas City, Missouri, met his wife-to-be Lauren on a blind date; five months later, they were engaged to be married. Then Lauren was diagnosed with breast cancer. During a routine MRI examination of her broken collarbone caused by a biking accident, doctors had found multiple tumors (the largest over 4 cm) in her breast. "I was speechless when I found out," according to Richard. "I wasn't sure what to say or do. We did not know how large the tumors were, how many there were, to what extent that it had spread, what kind of treatment would be best, what doctor(s) we'd need to consult, or her chances of survival. It felt as if a brick wall had just fallen on me."

Dr. Mary Jane Massie, a preeminent psychiatrist who specializes in psycho-oncology at Memorial Sloan-Kettering Cancer Center in New York City, describes the impact of a breast cancer diagnosis, "as if life has been shattered into prisms." To Marc Silver, author of *Breast Cancer Husband: How to Help Your Wife (and Yourself) through Diagnosis, Treatment and Beyond*, the diagnosis of his wife, Marsha, made him a member of a club that he never wanted to join. "When the news came . . . I became a breast cancer husband."

Your life forever changes when your loved one is diagnosed. Your life Before Cancer (BC) is gone—for good. You now live in the world After Diagnosis (AD). This is a world where control is not an option, where feelings of grief, guilt, anger, denial, fear, isolation, and anxiety collide inside you. After Diagnosis has swallowed you whole, and you are now in a black hole of misery, pain, numbness, shock, and nothingness.

When you heard the news, your initial response was probably one of complete disbelief. There is no way this happened to her.

There has to be a screwup in the results. They switched the films by accident. This isn't real.

So what the heck are you supposed to do now? Some medical health professionals recommend that you learn how to "manage" your emotions and get a hold of yourself. Get a grip, they say. Really?

Breast cancer isn't baseball. If it were, we could just ask Los Angeles Dodgers Manager Joe Torre to help us manage our "feelings" lineup: batting first and playing right field is Fear; batting second at shortstop is Anxiety; batting third and playing at first base is Isolation, followed by cleanup hitter Depression. Yeah, right. Since that doesn't work, perhaps a better way to begin is to better understand your opponent.

. . . .
What Is Breast Cancer, Anyway?
. . . .

Breast cancer begins when something goes wrong in a normal cell, a DNA mutation that affects other cells by multiplying, dividing, and then attempting to conquer healthy breast tissue. The earliest presence of breast cancer is known as DCIS, which stands for ductal carcinoma in situ. With DCIS, the cells have not invaded surrounding tissue. If these mutant cells continue to grow without treatment, they eventually form into a tumor. The size and number of tumors determine the "stage" of breast cancer. These stages are not finally determined until after surgery takes place, when the final pathology of the tumors happens.

Breast cancer is usually either ductal or lobular. Ductal means that the cancer arises from the ducts of the breast. Lobular occurs in the lobules of the breast. The aggressiveness of cancer cell growth varies drastically from one woman to the next. Frequently, tumors in younger women are more aggressive than those in older women who are not under the influence or control of estrogen. Like the staging process, the type of cancer cell that your loved one has is determined after a biopsy of the cells is made and the tissue is analyzed by an examining pathologist.

Most breast cancer cells grow slowly. Many invasive breast cancer tumors are present six to eight years before they are ever felt or seen during a typical breast examination. So the good news is that, in most instances, there is time to figure out the proper medical treatment for your loved one. The bad news is that you have plenty of time to think about all the bad things that could happen to her.

. . . .
What's Going to Happen to Her?
. . . .

Your first thought, and it's a natural one, is often this: is she going to die? It's the first question we all ask ourselves and that we must face. The good news is that in just about every case, the answer is a resounding NO! A National Cancer Institute study states that 89 percent of all women diagnosed with breast cancer are alive five years after their initial diagnosis. If the initial diagnosis occurs during early stage cancer, that number skyrockets to a survival rate of 98 percent.

The second question is: will she lose her breast or breasts? If the disease has been detected early, she has a 70 to 75 percent chance that her breast can be saved, thanks to a procedure known as a lumpectomy, which removes just the lump in the breast and preserves the rest of the breast. If the cancer has been diagnosed in early stages, survival rates for a lumpectomy procedure versus a mastectomy (complete removal of the breast) are the same.

The third question is: if you are her husband or boyfriend, what will breast cancer do to your marriage or relationship? Studies have revealed that divorce rates for couples in which the woman has been diagnosed with breast cancer are no higher than rates for other married couples.

It's all good, then, right? Not exactly. Statistics are just numbers, not guarantees. My mom, for example, swore to me that she would live to see my youngest brother, Kevin (who we call Bubba), graduate from high school. She never made it. A good friend of Sharon's didn't make it either, leaving behind three young boys and a grieving husband. In 2007, over 40,000 women died from breast cancer in the United States, according to the American Cancer Society. Indeed, it is the leading cause of death from cancer for women ages 15 to 54, and the second leading cause of cancer death for women ages 55 to 74, surpassed only by lung cancer. Women diagnosed at a young age, as well as women diagnosed with advanced-stage breast cancer at any age, are more likely to die from breast cancer than from all other causes of death combined, according to the National Cancer Institute.

Breast cancer is serious business. Unfortunately, today's high survival rates have lulled some people into a false sense of security. When Jenny of Virginia was diagnosed, her father didn't think it was important enough to go see her, from the time when she was diagnosed up until her final treatment. His thinking was that the survival statistics were so high that Jenny would be just fine. Well, she wasn't. She suffered a recurrence just one year later.

With that said, overall, the odds of surviving breast cancer are bright. Sure, breast cancer diagnoses are on the rise, but in the big picture, this is a good thing. Thanks to ever-improving detection equipment and medical knowledge about how breast cancer works, more and more women are being diagnosed earlier, which, when combined with ever-improving treatment regimens being developed, means more and more women will survive the disease. With five-year survival rates nearing 100 percent for women who are detected early, some medical experts have begun referring to breast cancer as a "treatable condition" instead of a disease.

The medical debate then turns to the ultimate question: will there be a cure for breast cancer discovered any time soon? Dr. Larry Norton, an internationally renowned oncologist and breast cancer researcher, has suggested that "a girl born today may not have to worry about breast cancer in her future." In fact, the number of research dollars targeted to finding a cure for breast cancer is staggering. The U.S. federal government, for example, spends over $900 million each year toward that goal. Millions more are spent by private industry and not-for-profit foundations. In 2007, the organization Susan G. Komen for the Cure donated $77 million for breast cancer research; it has contributed more than $450 million since its inception in 1982.

But all this talk is about the future of breast cancer treatment, not the here and now. Your loved one has just been diagnosed, and you need to help her, *now*. To begin the process of becoming a breast cancer caregiver, you need to better understand what exactly is going on in her head as she processes the idea that she has breast cancer.

What Is She Feeling?

The first, and certainly the heaviest, emotion that a woman experiences when told she has breast cancer is a fear of death. The implications are devastating. If she has a husband, she wonders how he will get along without her. If she has kids, she asks herself what's going to happen to them. If she is young and hasn't had kids yet, or has never even been married, she wonders whether she will ever have children—or a husband—at all.

The next emotional wave that washes over her after diagnosis is a feeling of loss. She feels that her health, independence, and happiness have all been unfairly taken away from her. Her anxiety increases with all the delays involved in getting the medical test results back. Most acutely, she feels a loss of control over her life—that her destiny is in the hands of others.

The longer she waits for results, the more she imagines the worst of outcomes. This growing anxiety leads to another significant fear: the fear of not being a woman. Women do everything, and more, that a man does in today's society, from heading Fortune 500 companies, to winning Nobel Prizes, to flying helicopters in Iraq, to running for president of the United States. But there's one thing she has that makes her different from all men, and that's her femininity. It's what makes her *her*. It's the way she dresses, the way she carries herself, the way she smiles, the way she smells, the way she acts, the way she tosses her hair, the way she bops down a street, the way she cries, the way she fights, the way she takes care of her family and friends, the way she laughs, the way she touches, the way she's touched, the way she kisses and hugs, the way she looks at you—and the way she looks to others.

In our image-obsessed society, the way she looks is a very big deal. The ideal woman is seen everywhere—on billboards, in magazines, films, television, and on fashion runways. We admire her face, her legs, her butt, and yes, her breasts. Men love breasts, and the media make sure we get our fill. The *Sports Illustrated* swimsuit issue, published in February every year, outsells every other issue the magazine prints by a factor of ten. In February 2006, for example, the *SI* swimsuit cover featured eight supermodels, all topless, and it sold over 1.2 million copies. When Victoria's Secret posted its first catwalk show on the Internet in 1999, over 1.5 million viewers tuned in, until the volume of viewers crashed the site. Victoria's Secret's bra models are all superstars, so well known that they are referred to on a first-name basis—Gisele, Tyra, Laetitia, Heidi. In 2002, with the first network television airing of Victoria Secret's Fashion Show, the event was seen by over ten million viewers.

In television and film, there are Angelina, Nicole, Naomi, Salma, Uma, Charlize, and Pamela. In music, there's Beyoncé (who, by the way, adorned the 2007 *SI* swimsuit cover), Britney, Madonna, Christina, Rihanna, Kelly, Nelly, Fergie, Ciara, Shakira. Then there's Janet, as in Janet Jackson, who infamously exposed her breast during a "wardrobe malfunction" while performing with Justin Timberlake at the February 2004 Super Bowl. Despite the fact that CBS received over 200,000 complaints about the incident, and received a $550,000 fine from the FCC for violating TV indecency standards (which was later overturned on appeal), Janet's breast exposure holds the distinction of being the highest replayed TiVo moment in history.

It's no wonder, then, that a survey in the women's magazine *Jane* revealed that 75 percent of women surveyed are unhappy with their breasts. "We don't often get to see what natural breasts look like," the writer of the magazine article claimed, thanks to the constant bombardment of "false images of 'perfection' that leave us feeling bad about ourselves." Imagine, then, the extreme emotional impact on a woman when she learns that she might lose one or both of her breasts, thanks to cancer. Her womanhood is on the line. Marisa Acocella Marchetto, author of *Cancer Vixen*, was a cartoonist for *The New Yorker* magazine when she was diagnosed. "My world came to an end," Marisa writes in her book. "The Electrolux of the universe sucked me into a Black Hole. I was alone."

What Is She Feeling as a Wife?

When my wife was diagnosed with breast cancer, Sharon's first thought wasn't about death, her career, or even her own children. It was about me, her husband, sitting next to her with a face frozen in sheer panic. She reached over, grabbed my hand, squeezed hard, and looked into my eyes. The first words out of her mouth, after the doctor had told her she had breast cancer, were to me: "I am so sorry."

She was *sorry* for getting cancer! She was sorry because my mom had fought breast cancer for ten years before dying from it. So Sharon wanted to make sure that I was going to be okay before she thought anything about herself. This was followed by a much stronger, and scarier feeling: would I still find her attractive? A wife's worst fear is that her husband is going to leave her, unable to deal with what one woman refers to as "damaged goods."

Nobody knows how many men leave a marriage after their wives have been diagnosed with breast cancer. What is known is that every patient reception area in the country has at least two or more juicy "bad husband leaving" stories circulating in it at any given time. Does a breast cancer diagnosis make men go bad? No. What it *does* do is exaggerate everything that's already been happening in a marriage—the good, the bad, and the ugly.

If you are a husband, the time has arrived for you to be on your best behavior since you walked down that aisle with her. What your wife wants from you most is for you to show up and be there for her. That's going to mean accompanying her to her appointments, helping her make her medical decisions (if she wants you to do that with her), comforting her, and the biggest thing of all—listening to her. After a diagnosis, the husband becomes the principal caregiver in the relationship. This role reversal is perhaps the greatest challenge placed on a marriage by breast cancer, and if you are her husband, it's up to you to be ready for that challenge.

What Is She Feeling as a Mother?

The greatest fear of every mom diagnosed with breast cancer is that of abandoning her children by dying. The younger her children are, the greater that fear. Annette from Texas was holding her nine-month-old baby when she got the news that she had breast cancer. "I sank to the ground, my daughter still in my arms, and started crying and crying. The baby, not sure how to take it, thought I was laughing, and so she proceeded to laugh and giggle at me." Annette refused to believe the diagnosis.

"My kids were just too damn young! That's what I kept saying to the doctors, over and over again. Are you sure it's me? This has got to be a mistake. And it *was* a mistake, until they showed me the tumor with my name right on the mammogram. The tumor was a really strange shape, like a dumbbell, with the smaller end ready to break off into another tumor. Then I got it."

When my wife went out to help my sister Mary in Arizona after my sister was diagnosed, all they could talk about were their children and how they had to be around for them, whatever the cost. My mom had the same fear when she was diagnosed in 1978. Back then, the doctors gave her just six months to live. She told her doctors she'd be damned if she was leaving her family that soon. Her doctors, shaking their heads, said the choice wasn't hers. She defied them, though, again and again. "She had kids to raise, meals to put on the table, laundry to wash, games to get the kids to, all those things a mom does," according to my dad, William ("Bill") P. Anderson Jr. "Cancer wasn't going to stop her."

What Is She Feeling as a Daughter?

My wife is a "daddy's girl," so to Sharon, her father was the hardest person of all to tell about her diagnosis. "When I told daddy, he dropped the phone," Sharon recalls. "I was crying so hard because I knew how much it hurt him. I was so hurt about what I had done to him. He was overcome with grief—so much so that he gave the phone to my stepmother to talk to me. He couldn't talk."

There is nothing more painful than to watch a parent struggle with the fear that his or her child might die first. That's because this scenario breaks the natural rule of the universe, and so it seems unfair—which it is. A father is often the first relationship a daughter has with a male in her life. It is from her father that a daughter begins to perceive herself as a female. And the impact that a father has on a daughter is so deep that scientific studies have shown its deep roots extend to when she begins puberty and how she develops as an adult. Perhaps the strongest feeling a daughter has toward her father, after she tells him about her breast cancer, is guilt. She then internalizes the pain she has caused him. Indeed, the pain and suffering a daughter feels when she tells her father that she has breast cancer is deep and long-lasting.

What Is She Feeling as a Sister or Friend?

I was raised in a family of six siblings—five brothers, and one sister, Mary. When Mary was diagnosed, she was afraid to tell me, because we had both gone through the pain and suffering of breast cancer with our mom. Her focus, toward me anyway, was one of protection: she didn't want me to be hurt again by what we had always referred to as the "Big C." At the same time, Mary knew that I understood the deep emotional and physical challenges breast cancer treatment entailed. She needed, in other words, her Big Brother—me—to be there for her, as her rock and confidant.

Every brother–sister relationship is different. Sharon was the older sister of two brothers. She wanted to know that her brothers would be there for her to make her laugh and forget, for a moment, the difficult journey that lay ahead for her. But many women today facing breast cancer don't have their families nearby to be there for them. Often, then, they turn to their friends and coworkers.

· · · · · · · · · · · · · · ·
What Are You Feeling?
· · · · · · · · · · · · · · ·

Sadness. Anger. Helplessness. Isolation. Grief. Numbness. Heartbreak. Guilt. Distraction. Pick your emotion, or emotional cluster—it changes on a moment's notice. "My heart goes out to men when their loved ones get the news that they have breast cancer," says Dr. Mary Jane Massie, a psycho-oncologist at Memorial Sloan-Kettering. "There is a tremendous burden on men to do the right thing." All this stress creates an abyss, which Henri J. M. Nowen, author of *The Inner Voice of Love,* describes as "a deep hole in your being." The abyss is a terrible feeling of aloneness, of being on the outside, not only with others but also with yourself.

In the early days of my wife's diagnosis, I suffered from a recurring nightmare, which scared the living daylights out of me. It was a hyperreal dream, in that everything in the dream took place inside my bedroom. The bedroom was exactly the same—the dresser, the bed, even where my wife Sharon laid next to me. But when I went to touch Sharon, in the dream she disappeared, as did the rest of the room. I went into a totally dark room, where no one could see or hear from me—ever again. When I awoke, I hesitantly touched Sharon, who, thank God, jumped up in fright and stared at me like I was a crazy person—which I clearly was. To me, the nightmare meant that I was afraid that breast cancer was going to take away not only my wife but me as well. Fear had me in its grip.

Anger is fear's terrible twin, which also often surfaces after a diagnosis. Guys are trained since we were little boys not to show fear, so we do what we think is the next best thing—get angry and take it out on someone else. Target number one for a man who has just been told that his loved one has breast cancer is the doctor—most specifically, the surgeon who has just announced her disease. Yet when you're angry, the worst thing that you can do is act out on that anger by screaming at the surgeon.

"I can't tell you how many men have screamed at me," said breast surgeon Dr. Beth Ann Ditkoff. "They need to act out because they simply can't deal with the stress. This is probably the most harmful thing a man can do for his loved one. As doctors, it's our job to get her better. The danger with screaming is that it could alienate the medical staff from doing its best job in helping her."

Next time you have to talk to a doctor about your loved one's breast cancer, check your anger at the door. Her doctors didn't give her the cancer; they just found it. They want to save her, not hurt her.

. . . .

Why Did This Happen?

. . . .

No one knows. Thousands of medical studies highlight the risk factors that "cause" breast cancer. There's obesity, high-fat diet, smoking, alcohol use, family history, lack of exercise, and so on. There are other statistics that weigh in as well, such as the age when the woman reaches puberty, age when she gives birth to her first child, and the age when she begins menopause. Then there are factors like whether she breast-fed her children or not, whether she even had children, and if so, how many. The list is endless—how tall is she, what is her height, what is her socioeconomic status, her ethnicity—on and on and on.

So why did your wife get breast cancer instead of the neighbor, coworker, best friend, sister, mother, grocery store cashier, bank teller, or doctor who told her she had it? The first "why" most people assign is because other women in the family have had cancer. That certainly seemed true with my sister, Mary. My mom had had breast cancer, as well as colon cancer. My dad had suffered from colon and prostate cancer. Then there were several great aunts who had breast cancer as well. In reality, though, the vast majority of women diagnosed with breast cancer come from families in which there is no family history—none at all—for breast cancer; that totals an estimated 80 to 85 percent of all breast cancer patients.

If medicine and statistics can't give us the definitive answer, maybe religion can. Rabbi Josh Zweiback of Congregation Beth Am in Los Altos, California, says that religion offers four classic responses as to why someone gets sick. The first is that the illness is a punishment by God, incurred because of something the sick person did. The second is that the illness is some form of atonement for past sins, perhaps for a bad thing a family member did years ago. The third reason is that God has imposed the illness out of love, that the illness comes out of an understanding of the true values and truths of the universe. Finally, there is the explanation that illness has no higher meaning at all, in that God is not the direct cause of suffering, and therefore cannot be held responsible for the illness. Rabbi Zweiback offers a unique, fifth religious meaning for why someone gets sick: that the illness is a test of how the caregiver responds to the sick person. Under Zweiback's theory, "the way we support and heal one another is an expression of our deepest beliefs about what God wants of us in the world."

Examining the same question from a Christian perspective, C. S. Lewis wrote in his journals that sickness is a test by God of faith— the faith not only of the infirm but also of the caregiver. Other Christian theologians believe that the answer to why sickness and pain exist in the world traces all the way back to Eve, who listened to Satan and got Adam to eat the apple, which led to their banishment from Eden—in other words, a woman's incredible pain suffered, say, at childbirth, was imposed by God as a punishment for eating from the tree of knowledge. So, would breast cancer pain apply under this theory as well? Surely not. The bottom line is this: there is no answer to the question "why?" So let's focus instead on something that *does* have a definitive answer for caregivers—what can we do for her? The best answer to this question is completely based on what your relationship is to her.

. . . .

What Can You Do as Her Husband?

. . . .

The first thing you can do is—nothing.

Huh? Doing nothing goes against every fiber of our being as men. We operate, quite well actually, when the rules of engagement apply: take business, sports, and war as three great examples. We have a mission, we make a game plan, and we execute. We seem to have a burning need to get things done—close a deal, wash the car, develop a new software program, pay the bills, run three miles on the treadmill in under thirty minutes. We're supposed to be doing something, always, all the time. And with breast cancer, there's so much that needs to be done—medical treatment decisions and scheduling; how and what to tell to family, friends and coworkers, and bosses; detailed conversations with insurance companies; and financial planning.

Well, all of this, and much more, needs to wait—for her. That's because you need to let her take the lead on what happens next, and when it happens. Nothing happens until *she* decides it is time to make something happen. The reason for this is simple: it's her body and her life that are under siege. Take your lead from her actions, not the other way around. The key here is to *react*, not act. The best advice comes from the great Chinese philosopher Lao-tzu: "the way to do is to be."

Your primary focus, as her husband, is to be there, physically and emotionally, in her moment of need. Never in your life will you have to show as much patience and restraint as at this moment of her initial diagnosis. Everything about who and what she is has been placed under severe attack. Her femininity has not only been called into question but is under threat of complete obliteration. Your role here is to remind her that everything is going to be okay and that you are there, just for her.

You are now the primary caregiver for her. Back when you first agreed to be her husband, you promised to be a caregiver if she ever got sick. Your wedding vows most likely said that you would be there for her, "to have and to hold, from this day forward, for better, for worse, for richer, for poorer, in *sickness* and in health, to love and to cherish 'til death do us part." The fascinating thing about this vow, which incidentally is derived from the Book of Common Prayer, is that the "in sickness and in health" phrase is the only sequence in the vow where the negative event is proclaimed before the positive one. Maybe that's because it's the hardest thing of all to do in a marriage.

How, then, do you begin to start taking care of your wife? Easy.

Listen. Listen. Listen.

You need to stop talking at her, or even with her, and just listen *to* her. Mirror her mood. If she wants to laugh, laugh with her. If she wants to cry and be afraid, comfort her and don't minimize her fear. If she's angry, validate that anger, and agree with her that this cancer thing really sucks. Watch for her emotions and follow them where they lead. But don't react to her emotions and cause conflict. Hear what she's worried about, what she is scared of, and what she needs from you. Only offer your opinion if, and when, she asks for it.

Your wife needs to feel wanted. The best way to make her feel wanted is to show her affection. If that affection gets more intimate, that's fine, too. It's good for her to know that you are still sexually attracted to her, but you shouldn't put any pressure on her at this time if she's not in the mood. You especially have to follow her lead when it comes to the bedroom. She needs to know you are there for her—as you promised you would be when you said those hallowed words, "for better or worse."

When you've convinced her that you are there for her, that you will be there for her, be sure to give her plenty of time with family and friends. Women are much better communicators than men. She is going to need to share her feelings and fears with others beside you, so give her that time and space to have those talks. Make your home a welcoming place for friends and family and help them show their support for your wife (provided, of course, this is what she wants). And if you sense that she wants private time with someone, be aware of that and quietly excuse yourself before she has to ask you to leave the room.

Your physical presence is important after diagnosis, especially when it comes to medical appointments. That's because four ears are better than two—always. She may not always hear all of what's being said, or necessarily understand everything. When you listen to the doctor, really listen, you'll probably hear information that she didn't that will be helpful to her later when she's thinking out her options.

When you go with her to see a doctor, take along a notebook to write down everything that you hear during each visit. If you aren't a good note-taker, then have your loved one ask the doctor if you can bring along a tape recorder. If the doctor says no, respect that decision. The last thing that you want is to have the doctor–patient relationship begin on a rocky start. There are a large number of medical decisions that need to be made. When you mix the emotions and stress that you and your wife are feeling in with the tsunami of information that the two of you are receiving, some of it naturally gets jumbled. Note-taking helps to eliminate this problem.

The bottom line is this: you need to be there for her, whenever and however she needs you. Let her know that you not only love her the same way as you did before the diagnosis, but more so. It's also important to tell her that you are still physically attracted to her as much as you were before she was diagnosed. Your mission is to protect and defend her femininity, and how she feels about herself as a woman. Your wife must know, on a deep emotional level, that she is your one and only. In other words, she is and always will be your trophy wife. You must become your wife's biggest cheerleader. You are riding on an emotional roller coaster. She, meanwhile, is aboard an emotional rocket ship. You are her rudder, and that rudder needs to be steady and true. The time has arrived for you to be her Mr. Big—being there, for her, for whatever she needs, whenever she needs it. This is not the time to be running off to the office, gym, or bar. This is the time to be a grown man, a real man, which means being her caregiver.

Her world, and yours, has been completely altered by this diagnosis. Nonetheless, many wives act like things are normal in order to keep some semblance of control over their lives. Continue to ask if there is something more you can do, even if it is the fourth, fifth, or sixth time you ask.

· · · · · · · · · · · · · · · ·

What Can You Do as Her Father?

· · · · · · · · · · · · · · · ·

Be her daddy. A woman faced with a diagnosis of breast cancer is really scared. Back when she was a little girl, when she got scared, she most likely turned to you to give her comfort and assurance that everything was going to be all right. Now that things aren't, she needs you once again.

My wife, Sharon, said that whenever there was a major thunderstorm in the middle of the night, she would bolt from bed, run down the hall, and jump into her dad's arms. Right after she was diagnosed, her dad rushed to be by her side. Nothing meant more to her throughout her treatment than the extraordinary effort her dad showed in working sixty-plus hour weeks as an optometrist, and then somehow managing to be by his daughter's side at least once every three weeks until her treatment was completed.

For many fathers, there is one huge obstacle to being there for their daughters: distance. Fathers today are often geographically separated from their daughters, and that puts being there physically in conflict with a job or other commitments, or requires money that may not be available. To remedy this situation, a father might set up a regular time to check in with her on the telephone, to let her know that he is still there for her, however and whatever she needs him to be. Fathers need to be a fountain of positive energy. This isn't easy to do, as my father-in-law Dr. Jack Rapoport can attest. "When Sharon told me she had breast cancer, I was devastated," Jack recalls. "Parts of my life that I once had were gone, and I could never get them back again."

The greatest difficulty that any father struggles with when he hears his daughter has breast cancer is the ultimate question: what if I outlive my daughter? It's every dad's worst nightmare. Children are supposed to outlive their parents, period. When parents age, it's the children who are supposed to be there to take care of them when they become ill, not the other way around.

Well, that is not how things always work out. So a father's job, at this stage in the game, is to be a good dad to her. Parents need to be parents. This does not mean, however, that parents revert to treating their daughters as if they were kids. She is an adult now, and must be treated as one. A parent's role is to listen, be supportive, and at all costs, avoid leading the discussion of the disease and telling her what to do. It is your love, support, and presence she is looking for, not your direction. To make suggestions about treatment is a big no-no, unless she directly asks for your help with this.

Dads, in the end, can empower their daughters by showering them with love, affection, and positive energy, and by supporting their daughters' decisions in treating the disease. Remember, she needs your shoulder to cry on. Dads, let her be your little girl again. It's okay. Take care of your little girl as only a great dad can do for his daughter. She needs to hear you say that you are there for her, however and whenever she needs you.

What Can You Do as Her Son?

Being a good son to your recently diagnosed mother is all about showing her the respect and dignity she deserves in her time of need. She has spent her life taking care of everyone else. She made sure everyone, and everything, ranked higher—before her and her own needs. With breast cancer, that situation changes. As her son, she needs your help.

The problem is that she won't ask for your help. It's a son's job, then, to step up and show her that not only are you there emotionally for her but you will also commit to being physically present for her. Never forget that all mothers are masters at the art of deception. They tell you, for example, that they don't want anyone to bother about them, especially when they are sick. My mom hated it when people treated her differently because she had breast cancer. The key word here is *people*, not *family*. She acted as if she didn't want her family around worrying about her either, but truth be told, the reality was just the opposite.

When my mom was diagnosed with breast cancer the first time, I bought her lies about how she wanted me to stay in school, get good grades, and not worry about her. I didn't see her until after she had had her mastectomy, and when I did lay eyes on her, she burst into tears. I had made a huge mistake. So, don't let moms fool you. They need their boys right there beside them, showering them with love and affection.

It's the little things around the house that you can do that will make a world of difference to her. Don't offer to clean up around the house—just do it. And expect that she may react in less than a positive way. I remember when I asked my mom what I could do for her. She told me to do some laundry, and in the middle of folding, she criticized me for everything that I was doing wrong—not putting the right colors together, folding things wrong, putting the clothes away in the wrong places. Did I do that bad of a job? No. Her criticism came from her frustration that breast cancer had taken away control of her life. So she took it out on me. Moms can revert to old patterns, treating their sons like young boys. A mom can do this to get a sense of control back into her life—so let her have that control. Don't fight back. In fact, embrace it, because it shows how she is fighting to get her life in order.

As a son, your role is one of support, not command. How and what she does for treatment is up to her, not you. It's all right to ask her about her condition, and how and what her doctors recommend doing to treat it. It's fine for you to help her research her condition to determine the best course of treatment. Just don't tell her what she has to do, or not do. The best thing you can do, as her son, is to be there for her throughout her treatment, in whatever way best helps her get through it.

. . . .

What Can You Do as Her Brother or Friend?

. . . .

The greatest value in a brother's love is the comfort it offers. Brotherly love is unlike any other form of love, because brothers often know their sisters better than anyone else, including parents. They grew up together, through thick and thin, which yields a deep understanding developed over two decades or more of sharing life experiences together. Often, that special thing a brother can offer his sister is humor. That's because a brother, better than anyone else, can get her to laugh—which is so important during the diagnosis stage. Things are serious enough, but you can get her to smile.

One way that I helped my sister laugh was by shaving my head into a Mohawk, and then going with her to her first chemo treatment. She shaved her head as well, and we dressed up like punk rock musicians. Every time we saw someone's jaw drop in astonishment, we laughed so hard that our sides hurt. Mary and I were just being kids again. It was funny, and better yet, we were having fun. Suddenly, breast cancer didn't seem so bad, which made things a lot better for her.

When my brother-in-law David came to visit my wife Sharon, he did his childhood "God" imitation to get her to lighten up. Leaning into an upstairs air vent, he lowered his voice to a level rivaling James Earl Jones's Darth Vader: "Sharon, this is God speaking. Make sure that you do not become a porn star after your operation by ordering breasts larger than your head." David turned every opportunity to talk with Sharon into a positive experience. He was truly her guardian angel.

A brother brings the ability to be his sister's friend. He knows what she is really all about, and how best to make her feel better about herself in this very trying time. He is on an equal plane with her, something that can never happen in a parent–daughter relationship. Likewise, he isn't encumbered with the deep issues of a husband–wife relationship. In fact, there isn't as much at stake in a brother–sister kinship, so free and unfettered communication happens more easily. He can just step in. That's exactly what my five brothers (Steve, Mike, Terry, Chris, and Bubba) and I did when my sister was diagnosed: she let us into her house to take care of her three boys, clean the house, and whatever else she needed us to do.

There is significant, positive affection and respect between a brother and a sister. There is acceptance of each other, a relationship that doesn't get bogged down in petty differences and conflicts.

That's because siblings, when they become adults, live different lives, usually in different locations, with different careers, different desires, but they acknowledge the validity of each other's lives.

"Brotherly" intimacy holds true for a woman's close friends as well. The true definition of a brother today, several recent studies have revealed, has less to do with biology and living arrangements and more with circumstances and experiences. Owing to divorce and separation, which create repartnering and extended stepfamilies, there may be a vast network of full, half, and stepsiblings, along with close friends, that your loved one considers to be her "brothers" and "sisters."

. . . .

What If She Has Children?

. . . .

If there are children at home, as there often are, they need to be told about their mother's diagnosis as soon as possible. When she is comfortable doing so, she should tell her children directly, with the husband standing right by her side for support.

Kids sense when something is wrong. After a breast cancer diagnosis, it is very hard, if not impossible, to hide the emotional tempest in the house created by the news. So it is vital to just be honest and explain the diagnosis at an age-appropriate level. Never lie to children about breast cancer. They instinctively know how bad things are. If you lie to them, telling them that it isn't as bad as it really is, the next time you tell them something, they won't trust you. Also, if information is held back, they imagine the worst will happen.

Again, what a child is told should be age-appropriate. The news may be a bit unsettling for a younger child; he or she may not be able to grasp in detail exactly what is happening to Mom. So, what you tell a five-year-old is different from what you share with a teenager. Tell each child individually, in private, where he or she can grasp the meaning and emotionally deal with the news. Let the child feel that he or she can do something for Mom. Maybe have the boy or girl draw a picture for the mother, spend time with her watching her favorite movie, make her something to eat, or perform for her by acting or playing music.

Older children can become great helpers at this time. More and more, young adults are moving back home after college. An estimated 34 percent of young adults live at home, according to Aaron Yelowitz, professor of economics at the University of Kentucky. It's important that these returnees contribute, rather than inhibit, her preparation for the fight. There's no hiding the fact that, in normal times, there is natural tension between parents and their adult offspring—in no small part because of differences in lifestyle. So, get them involved with household chores, such as cooking and cleaning; taking her to her medical appointments; and helping with younger siblings.

Who Else Should Know?

Most women diagnosed with breast cancer want their immediate family to know about the diagnosis. Exceptions to this rule certainly apply, especially when your loved one has strained relationships with one or more family members. Again, the best approach is to let her indicate who needs to be told, when that should happen, and how much information is divulged. Some women, for example, don't want anyone, including their own children, to know. This isn't recommended, however, since everyone is going to sense something is wrong by changes in mood, loss of hair, surgery, and the like.

As for those beyond the immediate family, there is no protocol for who is told. Some women will tell thirty people or more the first day they learn of their diagnosis, while others will not tell anyone, from initial diagnosis through final recovery. In most situations, a woman will probably want the information to be given to her friends in waves—closest friends first, followed by her next circle of friends, and then to neighbors and acquaintances. It will probably fall upon the caregiver to inform others outside of the immediate circle of friends, and the best way to do this is to tell each person in a quiet setting and explain that she is doing fine.

After the word gets out about the diagnosis, however, the next problem that often arises is an inundation of offers of help. It is common for friends and neighbors to bring food, offer to drive her to her appointments, phone or visit—whatever is needed. This bombardment of attention can have a countereffect, as most likely she needs time to herself and to be with her closest friends. A critical role for a caregiver, then, is to act as a gatekeeper, limiting access to those whom she wants most to be around her. You'll need to set limits; if the phone is ringing off the hook, be sure she is not being worn out by talking to too many callers—she'll need that precious energy and focus to sustain the treatment. Likewise, too many phone calls puts her in the position of having to repeatedly educate, console, and help calm everyone else's fears rather than her own.

One great way to keep everyone informed, while securing much-needed separation from a bombardment of "how are you doing?" questions directed at her is the Internet. There are many online sites that connect friends and family to the person who is sick, without invading her privacy. This is an especially valuable resource for friends and family who are not close by. The big three of these services are caringbridge.org, carepages.com, and thestatus.com. The *Los Angeles Times* reported that caringbridge.org has hosted over 61,000 sites for sick patients, while carepages.com has set up nearly 60,000 sites.

The real value of these sites is to eliminate false rumors and to supply the most up-to-date information about the patient without involving her. Information can also be provided as to the best times to call the patient. Since the sites are password protected, only those with the appropriate patient ID and password can enter. Contact information is provided, and guest messages can be left to show support.

Finally, there is the question of informing employers, both hers and yours. She will probably take time off during treatment, and you might need some time in the months ahead to help with that treatment. Almost everyone has seen either a family member or a friend go through breast cancer treatment, so most bosses are sympathetic to her and your needs. How much detail she shares about her condition depends on the type of person her boss is, as well as the corporate culture and its policy on sick employees. Most important, go to the boss as soon as possible, to assure that work is made more manageable during this crisis. The recommended way to talk with any boss, especially about breast cancer, is in private. This allows for open communication and greater comfort in discussing the subject.

···················· CHAPTER 2 ····················

Breast Cancer War

Assembling Her Armed Forces

BREAST CANCER CALLS for full-scale war. It's game on, every morning, every night, round the clock, every day, every week, every month, every year, for years to come. The battleground is her body, mind, and spirit, as well as your mind and spirit. The enemy is cancer, an overly aggressive, tireless foe committed to one mission and one mission only: to kill her. There's nothing greater at stake in her life—or yours. That's why her Armed Forces—her doctors, family and friends, spiritual guides, psychological advisers, and you—must be the strongest medical, emotional, mental, and spiritual team ever assembled to achieve the ultimate goal: stopping her breast cancer for life.

The term "Breast Cancer War" was coined in 1936, when the American Society for the Control of Cancer formed the Women's Field Army (WFA) to fight "trench warfare with a vengeance against a ruthless killer." By 1943, WFA members had swelled to over 350,000 strong. Today, powerful breast cancer organizations, like Susan G. Komen for the Cure, Breast Cancer Network of Strength, the National Breast Cancer Coalition, American Cancer Society's Reach to Recovery, and the Young Survival Coalition, to name just a few, have galvanized millions of women (and men) in the United States and around the world to raise billions of dollars for medical research to find a cure, and to provide the very best medical information and support for breast cancer patients and survivors. This "breast cancer sisterhood" is arguably the most powerful advocacy group for any disease—so strong, in fact, that the month of October is known as Breast Cancer Awareness Month.

The color of October is as much pink as it is the yellows and reds of autumn leaves. There are breast cancer walks (Avon Walk for the Cure), runs (Susan G. Komen's Race for the Cure), bike rallies (Bike 4 Breast Cancer), triathlons (Danskin Women's Triathlon Series), fashion shows (Fashion Targets Breast Cancer), parades (Parade in Pink), U.S. postage stamps (Stamp Out Breast Cancer), football games (NFL Breast Cancer Awareness Weekend), television movies (*Why I Wore Lipstick to My Mastectomy*), and countless public service announcements (e.g., Lifetime Television's "Stop Breast Cancer for Life"). Then there is the pink sea of product tie-ins: Lee jeans (Lee National Denim Day), M&M's (pink M&M's, and a pink M&M-branded race car for all NASCAR races that month), Campbell Soup (pink and white cans), KitchenAid (Cook for the Cure appliances), Tic Tac (Pink Ribbon Tic Tacs), Igloo (Pink Ribbon Playmate Pal Cooler), Sanyo (Always Pink Phone), Ford (Warriors in Pink Mustang), Rado (Time to Fight watch), Everlast (pink boxing gloves), Estée Lauder (Pink Ribbon Lipstick collection), Mattel (Pink Ribbon Barbie), and Ty Beanie Baby (SpongeBob Pink Pants). Even vacuum cleaner manufacturers have gotten into the act with the Dirt Devil Pink Rechargeable Broom Vac and the Dyson DC 07 Pink Upright Vacuum.

How do we guys fit into all this? Well, up to now, not very well. The moment when my wife became an official member of the breast cancer sisterhood, when her doctor said the words, "It's malignant," I was immediately separated from her. I was deposited in an "Information Room," filled floor to ceiling with "everything that you will need to know about breast cancer," according to the nurse who left me there, dazed and confused, encased in a mental sea of complete and total blankness.

What was I supposed to do? I had no idea. So I started to hyperventilate. The world began to spin. I couldn't breath. I sat down, and stared—at the paper: row after row of books, pamphlets, newsletters, and support-group meeting notices. What I remember most about that moment was that all the words on all that paper suddenly disappeared. I had been transported to a scary, fearful, dangerous, disorienting, alternate universe. I had been transported to Cancer Land.

It's hard to describe what living in Cancer Land is like until you place your feet on its *terra firma*. It sounds like a kid's game, like "Candy Land" or "Chutes and Ladders." But it is the farthest thing from anything even remotely related to fun. Cancer Land, for her and for you, is a place that initially fills you with feelings of sickness, fear, anxiety, helplessness, disorientation, worry, self-criticism, self-doubt, guilt, panic, nervousness, stress, nausea, headaches, depression, and isolation. It is truly a scary place—at first. But thanks to the millions of hardy souls who have already trekked this formidable land, there is great hope and promise that you and your loved one will not only successfully traverse Cancer Land but will also conquer it and claim it as your own.

Once you enter Cancer Land there is no turning back. If you try to turn around, there will be only failure and ruin for you and for her. So buck up and start moving forward by following your leader, your loved one. She is the one who presides over all things that happen—and will ever happen—in Cancer Land. She is your Alpha and your Omega, your beginning and your end, your Supreme Leader of all that lives and breathes in Cancer Land. She is your George Washington, Queen Elizabeth, Gandhi, Joan of Arc, Julius Caesar, Mother Teresa, Captain James T. Kirk, Rosa Parks, Rocky, your everything. She is your Commander in Chief.

· · · · · · · · · · · · · · ·

The Commander in Chief and Her Armed Forces

· · · · · · · · · · · · · · ·

The U.S. Constitution appoints the president as the country's commander in chief, the "Chief of the Army and Navy of the United

States, and of the militia of the several states." Likewise, cancer has anointed her as your commander-in-chief of Cancer Land. That's because it is *her* disease. She is the only reason Cancer Land exists at all. This gives her special privileges and responsibilities that no else has, or should have, or will ever have throughout the treatment process and beyond.

How and when your loved one executes her powers as commander-in-chief is always up to her, and never up to you (with the one exception being if she suffers from mental incompetence), regardless of your personal relationship with her as husband, father, son, brother, cousin, friend, or coworker—and especially as her ex-husband. She's in charge, period.

So what happens, you ask, if she doesn't act right away after the diagnosis in deciding her treatment options? Nothing. It is not unusual for a woman to be shell-shocked after receiving the news that she has cancer, and she needs time to process the emotional bomb that's just been dropped in her lap. In many, if not most, cases a few weeks' delay before beginning treatment won't hurt her future chances of survival. Patience, on your part, is critical here. It will show her how well you Stand by Her.

Every commander is different. Some women, like my wife, will take total control of everything that needs to be done medically. Other women will decide to put their complete trust in their medical team, and they don't want to know anything more after that selection is made. Then there is a third group that falls somewhere in between the two extremes. Whichever direction she takes, her powers are absolute in Cancer Land, at all times and in all instances. With that said, like every great leader, she must build around her a powerful and effective force—her Armed Forces—to overcome all the perils she will face to claim victory for her personal breast cancer battle. Just as the president of the United States relies on the Army, Navy, Air Force, and Marines to help him conduct his military operations, she must assemble and rely on what I like to refer to as her Medical Army, The Corps, Financial Navy, and Soul Air Force in Cancer Land.

. . . .

The Medical Army

. . . .

The battle against breast cancer begins, and ends, with medicine. Doctors make the initial diagnosis. Doctors perform the breast surgery. Doctors devise the chemotherapy regimen. Doctors do the radiation. Without doctors, the cancer battle would be over before it ever began. Good doctors fight breast cancer well. Better doctors fight cancer better. The best doctors fight cancer best. The better all her doctors work together, as a team, the better her chance for survival. The end result of this approach is the creation of a comprehensive treatment plan that is coordinated among the practice groups. Whatever decisions are made regarding the overall medical regimen, her medical team is on the front lines of the fight. That's all fine and good, you say, but how does she go about assembling that crack medical army? Well, it all starts with the selection of her breast cancer surgeon.

The Breast Surgeon

Think of a breast surgeon as the first five-star general of her army. As soon as her cancer has been identified as suspect, it is the breast surgeon who is called in to decide the critical next step. He or she makes the diagnosis with the help of the pathologist and performs the critical surgery from which all medical actions follow. The surgeon is responsible for removing her tumor or tumors, making sure that all the margins are clear, and ensuring that it doesn't come back; he also determines whether the cancer has spread to other parts of the body. The surgeon is the point from which all other medical team members emanate, ranging from the pathologist to the oncologist to the radiologist. It is the surgeon who oftentimes works at the crossroads of these specialties and who translates the medical language of those specialties for the patient and her caregivers. Indeed, the breast surgeon is the first of several five-star generals in the medical army, so your loved one wants to make darn sure she picks the right one.

Finding the Best Surgeons. The first thing she can do to find the best surgeon is to ask around, and the best place to start is with her primary physician; for many women, that doctor is her gynecologist. Her physician will have some great recommendations for a breast surgeon he or she likes best. The primary doctor, whether an internist or gynecologist, knows the patient's medical history intimately and, perhaps more important, has her trust. As you'll soon find out in this journey, being able to trust the treating doctors is critical. If your loved one doesn't trust her doctors, then there is real trouble in Cancer Land.

As soon as she gets a breast surgeon's name from her doctor, encourage her to book an appointment—immediately. Breast surgeons, especially the best ones, are booked solid. So the important thing, right away, is to get on that doctor's schedule. She can always cancel or reschedule the appointment, but the longer she waits to get on the books, the longer the wait to be seen and the longer to get her surgery scheduled.

It's also good to find out why the primary physician is recommending that particular breast surgeon. It can only help to know the specific medical reasons that surgeon is the top pick, so the more she can learn about the reasons for this recommendation, the better, and this entails finding out how informed her primary doctor is about surgeons. It's also a good idea investigate what direct experiences that primary doctor has had with other patients who have been referred to that surgeon.

A primary-care physician referral is just one of many ways to find the right surgeon, of course. Another great source is friends, family, and coworkers. If ever there were a time to draw on these resources, it is now. When my wife Sharon was initially diagnosed, we were amazed to think how many friends, family members, and coworkers she had whom she could call upon for help. Don't be afraid to tap friends of friends to get the name of the surgeon you want and need.

As mentioned, the more well respected the surgeon, the harder it will be to get onto that appointment calendar. An insider, someone who has access to or clout with that surgeon, can go a long way toward securing that golden ticket appointment. Call and e-mail everyone she and you know who could recommend a breast surgeon, and find out if they have an inside track to that surgeon as well.

Some times the patient herself has the inside track. My sister Mary's husband Joe, for example, worked at the Mayo Clinic in Scottsdale, Arizona, when she was diagnosed. It didn't take long, therefore, for her to get an appointment with any breast surgeon she wanted within the Mayo system. My wife, Sharon, tapped a married couple who were physicians at Columbia Presbyterian Hospital in New York City, who got her quickly through the door of her breast cancer surgeon, Dr. Beth Ann Ditkoff. Another great avenue for identifying the right breast surgeon for your loved one is to contact local hospitals in the area. That effort can begin with either a phone call to the hospital itself or a visit to the hospital's website. The website probably will not provide detailed information about a breast surgeon's credentials, but it will give basic contact information. With the surgeon's number in hand, contact the doctor's office directly and request a biography and brochure on his or her training, experience, and, if applicable, research done on breast cancer. It's not a bad idea to find out if the surgeon had a fellowship in breast surgery, and even more importantly, to find out if his or her practice is dedicated to breast disease, or is just a general surgery practice.

But don't stop there. She, or you, can go to the American Board of Medical Specialties (http://www.abms.org), where you can verify the breast surgeon's qualifications and certification; for example, that the doctor is board-certified. If you don't have Internet access, you can use the *Directory of Medical Specialists,* a huge reference book often available at your local library and certainly in the library of your local hospital. Further surgeon vetting includes contacting the state's medical board to check whether there are any lawsuits or disciplinary matters against that surgeon.

The Internet, of course, offers an overwhelming sea of choices, with countless "find a doctor" services. The basic level of these services usually provides free contact information. For a fee, you can obtain a more comprehensive analysis of a particular surgeon. Sites like healthgrades.com give comprehensive reports on targeted doctors, which include any malpractice actions, as well as a watchdog notification service and a physician-comparison report. These comparisons usually show years of practice, papers published, research conducted, and so on. Users of healthgrades.com can also buy a medical cost report that details the "total out-of-pocket expenses for a procedure," which includes "detailed cost estimates including procedure, drugs, and hospital stays." Other pay sites for similar searches include questionabledoctors.com, checkbook.org/doctors, and quackwatch.com.

Don't neglect to use the resources of her or your employer for a breast surgeon recommendation as well. At the corporate level, start with Human Resources; if the company is large enough, it probably has staff members who specialize in assisting employees with medical needs. Many large companies have access to medical reference services like Best Doctors (http://www.bestdoctors.com), a company started in 1999 by doctors from Harvard University School of Medicine, which provides a medical peer-review service with recommendations for the best doctors in various specialties across the United States. Likewise, check on any and all breast surgeons recommended by her insurance company, assuming of course your loved one has insurance. Whichever surgeon she ends up selecting, assuming money is an issue (as it is for most of us), it is always a good idea to make sure that her surgeon is included under her medical insurance policy. It should be noted that there are doctors, extremely qualified, who don't accept any insurance plans whatsoever because they have a large enough clientele to run a practice this way. If this is the doctor she wants to see, it's important that she have the financial resources to do so.

If all else fails, sheer perseverance wins the race to a great surgeon. Every surgeon, however high on the medical ladder that they stand, sees patients, so why not make that patient your loved one?

• • •

Throughout this book, I've stressed that the most popular patients for surgeons, oncologists, radiologists, and plastic surgeons are those who are well informed, persistent, passionate, and compassionate about what their doctors go through every day. So if she can put that personal package together, and successfully navigate the surgeon's protective maze of appointment secretaries and nurses, then there is no reason she can't move to the top of the list of the best surgeons available to her. Sharon, wanting to get to see a particular breast cancer specialist, sent a handwritten card to him; the card, having a "personal" look, passed right by his administrative gatekeepers. On the card was a picture of Wonder Woman opening the jaws of a giant monster, and inside Sharon asked, teasingly, what it would take to get this doctor's attention. He called her the day the card landed on his desk.

Stepping to the front of the line with her medical team is one of the most important things, if not *the* most important thing, your loved one can do for herself. A great way to make that happen is for her to get them to love her. Yep, you read that right. She needs to get love from her doctors. She must win the Best Patient contest over her fellow breast cancer patients. Keep in mind that it's not that the doctors don't care about their other patients; they do. It's just that doctors are human, like the rest of us, and like us, they have favorites. So why not make your loved one the favorite? The more her doctors care about her, the better they will take care of her, thereby giving her a greater chance of winning her cancer battle.

So, the more positive energy shown by the patient to her doctors, the more positive energy will be reflected right back to her by her medical team. The end result of all this patient/doctor "love energy" is an astounding amount of trust, which is critical in dealing with all the future uncertainties and fears.

The patient's interest in the different medical treatments shows her doctors an appreciation of the complexities and pressures they face daily in fighting breast cancer. If the patient doesn't have that curiosity, then maybe you, as her caregiver, can step forward as her shining light of medical knowledge. The more she, or you, know about the latest in breast cancer treatment, the harder her doctors will be pushed to implement those treatments to cure her. Another great tip in helping her become the Best Patient is to make sure she is always on time for her appointments, is organized with her questions, listens to what the surgeon has to say, is thoughtful about what he or she is trying to do, and is thankful for the effort.

Questions to Ask, Things to Consider. However her breast surgeon is found, make sure the surgeon meets your loved one's particular needs and specifications. Sharon wanted a breast surgeon who was smart yet caring, had a good reputation, was affiliated with a good hospital, was current on the scientific information and medical procedures, was willing to answer questions, and was open to being challenged—by her, the patient.

A critical requirement for any breast surgeon is that he or she has expertise in breast cancer surgical procedures. The quickest way to determine this is to examine the doctor's surgical "outcome measurements"; translated, this means finding out the number of mastectomies and lumpectomies that the surgeon performs each year, and then checking on the "complication rates" of infection—in essence, how many surgeries went bad. If your loved one is having a lumpectomy, it's good to review the surgeon's excision percentage rates.

As mentioned earlier, your loved one should make an appointment with a breast surgeon as soon as possible. Before the actual appointment, though, she needs to make sure that all the necessary films and pathology reports are sent to the surgeon for review beforehand, as well as confirm that the surgeon doesn't require additional reviews by radiologists or pathologists. Before entering the examining room, she should have a list of questions to ask the surgeon, prioritized in case all those questions can't be answered in one visit. Ideally, all of her questions will be answered during her initial visit, but just to make sure, she should get an assurance from the scheduling assistant that she will have the time she needs to ask all her questions and get the answers. The Boy Scout "Be Prepared" motto is never more applicable than when meeting with a breast surgeon. She should ask if the doctor is receptive to receiving e-mail questions before she arrives for the examination. If that's the case, then time spent with the surgeon will be more efficient for both parties. But, as breast surgeons are very busy people, her surgeon may or may not agree to this.

As for the questions themselves, the key is to put the most important ones front and center. Here are just a few suggested questions that can help her decide if the breast surgeon is right for her:

- What procedure do you want to perform on me?

- Why was this procedure chosen?

- What are the pros and cons of this procedure?

- How often have you performed this procedure?

- What have been the usual results of this procedure, and what can go wrong?

- What can be expected in post-op?

- What are the other surgical options besides the recommended one, and what are the pros and cons of these alternative procedures?

- How is the surgical site marked for the plastic surgeon and radiologist (if radiation is needed)?

- Are there any pictures or videos available to see the procedure or procedures being discussed?

The initial consultation leads up to one final, vital question: can she trust her breast surgeon? That is, is she willing to turn her body over to that surgeon to save her life? She must have confidence in not only the surgeon's technical skills but also in his or her knowledge of breast cancer treatment. It isn't a bad idea, then, for her to also ask what conferences the surgeon attends and how often, or if the surgeon has ever been invited to speak at these conferences or present a paper. It doesn't hurt to ask if the surgeon has been published in a medical journal, either.

When she gets closer to making her decision on a surgeon, your loved one needs to make sure that the selected surgeon is the one, indeed, who will do the actual surgery and not another surgeon in that medical group (which is what happened with Sharon when, at the last minute, the surgeon she wanted wasn't available, and she opted to go with the fill-in surgeon).

In deciding to go with one surgeon over another, it doesn't hurt for you and your loved one to observe how that surgeon treats his or her staff—whether it's engaging, dismissive, or somewhere in between. The more engaged the nurses are in the surgeon's work, the more interest they will take in your loved one's situation and the more care she can expect from the staff.

Both the patient and you, or whoever might be accompanying her to meet with the surgeon, should bring along pen and paper to write down the surgeon's responses. As mentioned earlier, it's always good for her to bring along a family member or friend, since four ears are better than two. It isn't a good idea, however, to have more than one person accompany her, lest there be too much distraction, for the patient as well as the surgeon. Expect that some time during the course of the appointment there might be interruptions, especially if the surgeon is in high demand. This can throw off the patient's, and your, train of thought and result in not having all the questions answered. So it is important to ask her most important questions first, and if all her questions are not answered by the end of the visit, to ask the doctor if there can be a follow-up visit or if a phone call can be scheduled to get the rest of her questions answered.

One way to ensure that she understands everything the surgeon has said is to tape-record the conversation, but as tempting as this is, it may not be advisable, and here's why. The physical presence of a tape recorder establishes a formal setting for the doctor–patient relationship at a critical time when both parties are just getting to know each other. The doctor, as well as the patient, might be overly concerned about what he or she says, inhibiting free dialogue. In fact, the tape recorder can make the visit feel more like an interview, turning the appointment into a stilted and inhibited experience.

Available Options. After the patient has undergone the initial examination by the breast surgeon and hears the surgeon's recommendation, she should inquire about other surgical options and observe how well the surgeon knows about alternatives and how solid that surgeon's medical reasoning is. Currently there are two standard approaches to breast cancer surgery. The first is lumpectomy, which is the removal of just the tumor itself, leaving the rest of the breast intact. The second is mastectomy, which involves full removal of the breast, or breasts. Whether a surgeon recommends a lumpectomy or mastectomy depends on the circumstances of the tumor or tumors— their size, number, type, aggressiveness, as well as her actual breast size.

A great place to learn more about the surgical decision-making process is *Dr. Susan Love's Breast Book*, now in its fourth edition, or reputable websites like those of the National Cancer Institute (NCI; http://www.cancer.gov); Breast Cancer.org (http://www.breastcancer .org); American Cancer Society (http://www.cancer.org); or any of the sixty-three NCI-designated Comprehensive Cancer Center sites in the country, which include Johns Hopkins, Arizona Cancer Center, Dana Farber/Harvard Cancer Center, Fred Hutchinson/University of Washington Cancer Consortium, and M.D. Anderson Cancer Center.

In deciding whether to have a mastectomy or lumpectomy, Dr. Susan Love, in her *Breast Book,* says that the decision rests entirely with the patient and not her loved one. "Husbands and lovers come and go, but your body is with you all your life," Dr. Love says. "A truly caring mate will support whatever course you think is best for you."

It is strongly recommended that, even after your loved one has narrowed her selection to one breast surgeon, she meet with another surgeon to get a second, unbiased opinion on treatment options. Ideally, the second surgeon will not be in the same practice or even in the same hospital system. Getting a second opinion certainly is an added expense, but it provides her with that feeling of security that comes from exploring all options. Barron H. Lerner, a medical historian and physician at Columbia University College of Physicians and Surgeons in New York City, attributes the concept of second opinions to headstrong breast cancer patients in the 1970s who "armed with growing knowledge of treatment options pressed physicians for information," despite oftentimes facing "patronizing dismissal" from their doctors. My mom, diagnosed in 1978, certainly faced her share of patronizing physicians. To counteract their condescension, Mom would clown with her doctors, literally, by putting on circus makeup, clown shoes, pants, fuzzy hair, nose, the works—when she walked into their offices. Her reasoning was, how could anyone argue with a cancer clown with nothing to lose? She was right. They backed down immediately and answered any questions she had.

If there are complex issues involved with the surgery, it is always wise for her to get a second opinion from another breast cancer surgeon. In fact, the only reason not to get another opinion is cost, either because the patient can't afford it or her insurance company refuses to cover it. If the latter is the case, then she can appeal the insurer's decision, which many times results in an overturned decision and subsequent approval for a second opinion.

For my wife, the second opinion saved her life. Her original surgical team found only one lump, so they recommended, and did, a lumpectomy. After the surgery, the CAT scan results showed that the margins around the tissue that had been removed were not clean, and so she would need additional surgery to remedy that problem, which can happen due to microscopic disease seen by the pathologist. Before going back to her original surgeon, Sharon got a second opinion from the Columbia Presbyterian Breast Center (now known as the Breast Center at New York–Presbyterian/Columbia). Dr. Beth Ann Ditkoff insisted that her radiologist, Dr. Marc Brown, review Sharon's films before Dr. Ditkoff saw her—after all, there is nothing wrong with a fresh medical look at a patient's scans. Dr. Brown found a second tumor on the edge of her scans that had been missed by the first examining radiologist. This important discovery of a second tumor, which proved to be cancerous, led to the recommendation for a mastectomy. It is hard to imagine the damage that a second tumor would have caused if it had gone undetected. "A second imaging evaluation is a must if the first evaluation is not thorough," according to Dr. James Mullett, a radiologist at the Carilion Clinic in Roanoke, Virginia. "This may include repeat mammograms, additional biopsies of suspicious areas, and [an] MRI, which is key to an assessment of the extent and distribution pattern" of the cancer.

To better help with the decision whether better care is behind Doc Number One's or Doc Number Two's door, your loved one should get recommendations, and discouragements, from patients who have been treated by those surgeons. Their offices will cite patients who have had positive experiences, but how can she find the naysayers? One way is through patient-support groups like Susan G. Komen and Reach for Recovery. Another is to turn to family, friends, and coworkers for names. If she belongs to a social or church organization, that might also be a source of patient names.

• • •

Should your loved one be treated by a surgeon who is part of a regular hospital, or by a surgeon associated with a medical school and/or a comprehensive breast cancer center? For the patient to make the best decision for herself, she needs to consider her initial diagnosis and the surgical recommendations. If the diagnosis is of a "standard" case of breast cancer (noting that cancer is never ever "standard," given the complexity of the disease), then a patient would be fine with a local doctor, provided that surgeon has performed multiple breast cancer surgeries.

If, however, your loved one's diagnosis requires advanced treatment, then the question becomes whether it makes sense for her to be treated at a university hospital or a National Cancer Institute—designated a Comprehensive Cancer Center (CCC). CCCs, scattered throughout the country and usually in major metropolitan areas, were established by the National Cancer Institute as teaching hospitals, equipped with the latest and greatest research, equipment, and techniques. In essence, they push the envelope in breast cancer care. If your loved one lives in a large city, chances are there will be a CCC nearby. But for patients outside of metropolitan areas, a CCC is probably not close. It should be noted that there are many qualified doctors outside the university and CCC systems who have advanced breast cancer surgical experience as well. The important thing to remember is that whoever your loved one ultimately chooses for her medical team, they need to be able to work in a coordinated fashion, even if they practice under different medical roofs. My wife, Sharon, for example, chose a surgeon who practiced in one hospital, an oncologist in another, and a radiologist in a third system, but they all worked very well together as Sharon's breast cancer treatment team.

So the decision on who to go with is a balance between treatment options, expertise, and convenience. Rare and aggressive cancers may call for treatment by specialists in that particular form of breast cancer. Two such rare forms of breast cancer are inflammatory breast cancer and Paget's disease. My mom had inflammatory breast cancer, named for its symptoms of a reddish rash that spreads across a woman's breast, causing unusual warmth to the skin. Paget's disease appears as a crusty, scaly buildup around the nipple that never gets better. But even if her cancer is typical, the better the medical team, the better the hospital, the better her chances for survival, so she should always stretch for the best of the best to treat her disease.

Thus, the most important step a woman can take in treating her breast cancer is to get the correct treatment for her disease. Recognizing that the success of her surgery, and of subsequent treatment, can't be determined until years later, she needs to get the best care she can find, anywhere. Recurrence is what every breast cancer patient fears most, so getting the correct treatment the first time is crucial to long-term success.

Bonding with the Breast Surgeon. It is critical that there is clear communication between the breast surgeon and the patient. Your loved one needs to know everything that is going to happen to her, as well as all her surgical options. Breast cancer is different from many other diseases because it directly attacks her femininity. With surgery, she faces the loss of part or all of her breast or breasts, depending on her diagnosis. She needs an expert in breast surgery, but because of the deeply emotional components of breast cancer, she also needs empathy and compassion from her surgeon. Dr. Ditkoff, my wife's surgeon, held Sharon's hand right up until the anesthesia took hold. When Sharon cried during a consultation, Dr. Ditkoff got up from her desk to hug her. There is absolutely nothing wrong with having a surgeon who makes the patient feel nurtured while still being professional and appropriate. But not every patient wants the same fuzzy-wuzzy treatment. Some patients feel uncomfortable with physical contact from a doctor. Whatever works best for the patient is what the doctor should do, for patients' needs should always come first. Touchy-feely might not be the best medicine for your loved one; instead she might want her doctor to be reserved and removed, concentrating solely on the medicine and not her emotions.

Doctors are getting increasingly emotionally involved with their patients. At a meeting before the Society of General Internal Medicine, Dr. Anthony D. Sung, of Harvard Medical School, claimed that 69 percent of medical students and 74 percent of interns have cried at least once in front of patients. This has sparked criticism as improper behavior in some medical circles, who call for a certain level of detachment to protect those doctors from "emotional burnout."

According to my wife, Sharon, physicians who take a more emotional approach give patients "an extra appreciation for doctors who feel comfortable with outward displays of emotion. If that means tears, bring it on." I'll never forget when a doctor cried openly in front of Sharon, after that doctor had successfully resuscitated our oldest son, Seth, at birth. Seth was not breathing when he was born, and his heart had stopped. Our son's neonatologist, Dr. Mary-Joan Marron-Corwin, was able to revive Seth by sticking an oxygen tube into his belly button where his umbilical chord had been attached just moments before. It turned out that Dr. Marron-Corwin had gone through the exact same procedure with the birth of her own son just a few weeks before. Everything turned out well for Dr. Marron-Corwin and her child; for us, the first twenty-four hours of Seth's newborn life would determine whether he would lead a healthy normal life or have brain seizures and permanent brain damage from lack of oxygen during this brief time when he was not breathing. The next morning, Dr. Marron-Corwin came into the room with wonderful news: our baby was going to be just fine. The vigil over, we could go home with a healthy, happy, newborn baby. When Dr. Marron-Corwin saw the fear in Sharon's eyes dissipate into a puddle of tears upon hearing the good news about our baby, she burst into tears as well. Doctor and patient hugged each other, as only thankful mothers do after facing a grave threat. Observing this exchange from the other side of the room, I considered it the most powerful display of care and concern from a doctor to a patient possible.

I don't remember Sharon's breast surgeon ever crying, but I never doubted that she cared for Sharon. Dr. Ditkoff had an intense attentiveness to detail, but was comforting at the same time. She never broke eye contact when talking to Sharon, or me. She had a rapid-fire way of acknowledging what she heard you say, a rat-a-tat of "uh-huh, uh-huh, uh-huhs" that resulted in the right answer to every question we asked. Sharon was constantly reassured by Dr. Ditkoff's ability as a surgeon, in no small part because her surgeon's mind traveled at the speed of light, confident in her ability—which, eight years later, is one of the main reasons Sharon is alive today.

The Diagnostic Radiologist

Unlike breast surgeons, with whom we expect, and often demand, compassion, a radiologist often never meets the patient. Yet it is the radiologist who finds the cancer tumors. I like to refer to these doctors as the eyes of God, a physician best described as the wizard behind the green curtain. The diagnostic radiologist often becomes part of the medical team by circumstance, having been the first to identify the tumor.

With that said, the relationship between a surgeon and a radiologist is critical. Many breast surgeons today will not operate on a patient unless their chosen radiologist has examined the tumors in question. Indeed, many teaching and research hospitals require that no surgeon on their staff operate without an internal review of the patient's scans by its hospital-affiliated radiologist.

The goal for the patient, then, is to make sure that the diagnostic radiologist has all the defining traits of a specialist in the field— namely, that he or she is accurate, methodical, definitive, focused, with an incredible eye to find not only tumors but even the most minute traces of cancer cells.

So how does one go about picking a diagnostic radiologist when they make themselves difficult, if not impossible, to meet? There are the same routes to selection as described above for finding a breast surgeon—personal referrals, physician recommendations, Internet research, hospital and insurance company suggestions, and the like—but perhaps the best route is to go with the radiologist your surgeon trusts the most. The closer doctors work together as a team, the better the chances your loved one has of killing her cancer.

The Oncologist

The oncologist is the doctor in charge of treating your loved one, usually after surgery; the doctor who makes sure that the cancer is killed not only in her breast but also throughout her body with medications—chemotherapy, biological treatment, and antiestrogen drugs. The oncology protocol is often not finalized until after breast surgery has been completed, when a pathologist has properly analyzed the tumor or tumors. As with breast surgeons, it is advisable for the patient to get a second opinion on what the best oncology regime should be.

Sharon, through her Superwoman efforts, was able to get not one, not two, but six oncologists to review her case and weigh in on the best course of treatment. Each oncologist's terms and conditions for the review were different. Some demanded that the pathology slides be sent so that their own team of pathologists could review them; other oncologists reviewed the original pathology reports and gave their opinions based on those reports. The good news was that five out of the six oncologists agreed on the same protocol for Sharon. The lone dissenter claimed that the best course of action was a stem cell transplant. It turned out that this oncologist was conducting research on the effectiveness of stem cell transplants as an oncology treatment and she needed more participants for her study. Sharon, smartly, didn't want to be that doctor's guinea pig and declined.

Leaving no stone unturned, Sharon even worked her magic to reach out and get an opinion from renowned breast cancer surgeon Dr. Susan Love. A physician friend of Sharon's was going to an international breast cancer medical conference where Dr. Love was speaking. He offered to take Sharon's pathology reports along with him, which he carried with him in his back pocket during the conference so that if he got an opportunity to ask Dr. Love if she would give an opinion about how Sharon should proceed with her treatment, he could hand her the report.

About a week later, while she was cooking dinner with her two boys fighting in the background, the phone rang. Sharon picked up the phone, and because of the noise, only heard the caller identify herself as "Susan." Knowing a large number of Susans, Sharon couldn't figure out which of her friends had called, and about what, since she could barely hear her over the shrieking voices of our boys. Everything changed, though, when she heard this Susan start talking about the path report. It was *the* Susan, Dr. Susan M. Love.

"I freaked out, running from the kitchen to my upstairs office where I kept my files which had every question that I ever wanted to ask her," Sharon recalls. "As I was desperately trying to find my questions, she had to wait, so to fill the time I said 'you know, three months ago, before I got diagnosed, the only person that I would have gotten this excited about to talk to on the phone would have been Mick Jagger. And now, here I am, just as excited to talk to you, Dr. Susan Love, about breast cancer. Oh, how the mighty have fallen!'" Dr. Love's response? "She broke into a big belly laugh when I said that."

Sharon then proceeded to ask Dr. Love every question that she ever wanted to ask. "Dr. Love was unbelievably patient and incredibly generous of her time, answering every question that I had, in detail, and then weighing in with her own personal opinions on everything to do."

● ● ●

The best chance to defeat breast cancer for life is to find it early, remove it quickly, and then eliminate any stray cells. The best oncologists are those who understand the risk–benefit equation that goes with all chemotherapy treatments. Finding the right oncologist requires the same vetting process as finding the surgeon discussed earlier in this chapter. This vetting includes getting recommendations through various networks of doctors, friends, family, and coworkers. It means looking into an oncologist's qualifications, including years of experience, success rates in treatment, research work (if any), and available data from patients and doctors. It is always a good idea to make sure the oncologist is board certified to practice chemotherapy, a fact that can be confirmed either through state medical boards or via the Internet. It is also critical that the oncologist be someone your loved one can afford, through private insurance, Medicare, Medicaid, or out-of-pocket payments. It could be argued that the oncologist pick is more important than the surgeon, since it is the oncologist who is going to be examining and treating your loved one for the rest of her life.

There is one big helper in the oncologist selection process: there is the breast surgeon's recommendation. For this reason, your loved one should follow through on that recommendation and learn more about that particular oncologist. This in no way means that your loved one has to take that recommendation. The choice of an oncologist is totally up to her, and her alone.

For a list of oncologists, your loved one can turn to the American Society of Clinical Oncology (ASCO), which has over 25,000 oncologists in its database, arranged by name, institution location, and board certification (go to http://www.cancer.net/portal/site/patient, then click "Find an Oncologist"). Additional places to look are the American Board of Medical Specialties database (http://www.abms .org) and the American Medical Association Doctor Finder database (http://webapps.ama-assn.org/doctorfinder).

Before making the oncologist selection, the patient should visit the treatment centers where her short-listed oncologists practice. She should see the setting where her treatments will be and imagine herself being there, receiving those treatments. She should talk to the nursing staff, and determine how knowledgeable they are on the latest treatments, the drugs and biologics being used, and how to deal with the side effects. She should find out whether the nurses are specialists in chemotherapy (which is highly recommended) by being an oncology certified nurse (OCN). She should talk to the patients about how they feel they are being treated. It's helpful, also, to find out if there is a social worker or psychologist in the practice who can help her, if needed, with emotional and psychological problems she and her loved ones might face as treatment proceeds.

It is vital that the patient like her oncologist. There is going to be tremendous emotional and psychological turmoil involved with the chemotherapy, so she needs to know that she can lean on her doctor when the going gets rough. Therefore, at that initial consultation, she needs to ask the best questions that will help her pick the right doctor. Much depends on the cancer diagnosis, but here are ten suggested questions for your loved one to ask:

1. What type of tumor(s) do I have, including its (their) hormonal status, and how does this affect the treatment regimen?

2. What are my chances that cancer will return—how will that be monitored, and how often, after all the treatments are completed?

3. What chemotherapy regimen (drugs, treatment sequence) do you recommend, and why?

4. What alternative chemotherapy treatments are available, and what are the advantages/disadvantages compared to the first recommended therapy?

5. What are the side effects and risks of the various chemo treatments, including but not limited to heart and bone damage, hair loss, nausea, tiredness, sleeplessness, stomachaches, lowered immunity, higher skin cancer risks?

6. What will the drugs/biologics do to my body, such as early menopause, osteoporosis, and infertility? How will it affect me mentally and emotionally?

7. What can I expect, in terms of disruption of work and home life, as a result of these recommended treatment options, and what is your plan to limit these disruptions?

8. How will the treatments affect me sexually?

9. How available will you [the oncologist] be before, during, and after each treatment?

10. What clinical trials are available for me and why or why should I not consider participating in one?

I want to revisit, for a moment, the consideration of a clinical trial for your loved one. She should always ask her oncologists being interviewed what clinical trials are available to her, not only in their practice but throughout the region, and around the country as well. She might qualify for a clinical trial of a new treatment that could one day save her life. For example, I am convinced that the clinical trial involving the drug Herceptin, used for early-stage cancer patients—a trial that my wife qualified for and participated in—saved her life. Sharon's oncologist, Dr. Suzan Merten, agrees: "For Sharon, she was very fortunate because she got on a trial that just proved to be earth-shattering wonderful news." Dr. Merten is a strong advocate for participation in clinical trials for breast cancer chemotherapy, not only because she is an oncologist but also because she is a breast cancer survivor. "When you talk about a clinical trial in the setting of a curable breast cancer, postoperative therapy for breast

cancer, there is no way breast cancer patients are guinea pigs, because there is no such thing as a clinical trial that won't at least
include all the drugs we [already] know that work. And what they
are doing in the clinical trials is just moving a step forward . . . by
either adding another drug to see [if it] will add to long-term survival, or take out a drug because . . . [it has] less long-term toxicity."

The Radiation Oncologist

Whenever radiation was mentioned in connection with my loved
one's cancer, it always made me think of some dark and dingy room
with huge metal equipment that shot out glowing green bolts of
light. The vibe was Dr. Frankenstein meets the Manhattan Project.
But the truth is that radiation oncology treatment centers are just
the opposite: bright, cheery places that bring comfort and hope.
Radiation as a treatment regimen for cancer has been around for
decades, and is an incredibly effective method for treating breast
cancer today.

When my wife was interviewing radiation oncologists to decide
who would be the best for her, she narrowed her selection to two
candidates. The first was a doctor who worked in Westchester
County, New York, in an office with a panoramic view of the Hud-
son River. In his waiting room, he had classical music softly playing
and a gigantic saltwater fish tank filled with lionfish, butterfly fish,
parrotfish, and groupers (can you tell I'm a scuba diver?). There was
a coffee bar in one corner and the magazines in the rack were up-to-
date. Despite feeling as if you were visiting a top-shelf country club,
there was a bit of coldness to the staff, which seemed at times hard
to shake.

The other doctor worked at White Plains Hospital in White
Plains, New York. This office was in the basement, so the look was
pure white, all minimalist. While the atmosphere was stark, the
personnel were the warmest that my wife encountered throughout
the process. The radiologist, Dr. Randy Stevens, smiled often and

had every answer possible for Sharon at the ready. The basement team won the race.

The Plastic Surgeon

The type of breast surgery that a patient receives determines if a plastic surgeon is part of your loved one's Medical Army or not. If she is getting a lumpectomy, probably not; if she is getting a mastectomy, in almost all cases, yes. For a mastectomy, the plastic surgeon usually begins reconstructive surgery immediately after the breast surgeon has removed the breast or breasts. This is best for the patient, because it keeps her time in the surgical room to one, and not two, visits. The exception to this rule is if the patient has positive lymph nodes, meaning the cancer has spread to her nearby lymph nodes, which usually means she will undergo radiation therapy. In this case, it is sometimes recommended that she postpone reconstruction surgery until after the radiation therapy is completed.

As with all the other members of her Medical Army, it is important for your loved one to feel comfortable with her plastic surgeon. That comfort ultimately comes from the work the plastic surgeon does in breast reconstruction. Today, patients choosing a plastic surgeon can see, firsthand, the plastic surgeon's past work. They can, for example, get an actual "feel" by touching another woman's breasts that have been reconstructed by that plastic surgeon. As crazy as this sounds to us guys, women do it all the time. My wife felt a pair. She touched the reconstructed breasts of my mom's best friend, Caryl. Here's how the conversation went, in a women's clothing store, right between a rack of sweaters and blouses, as a fellow female shopper stood by, listening and watching in shock:

CARYL [grinning]: "You wanna feel them?"

SHARON: "Really?" Caryl nods. Sharon, tentatively, reaches out and touches Caryl's breasts.

SHARON: "Wow . . . they are . . ."

CARYL: "Firm, right?" Sharon and Caryl laugh, while the woman in shock shakes her head, and walks away.

So, plastic surgeons have a unique ability to show off their work. In addition to actual results, they can show before-and-after photos of patients they have treated.

The image of plastic surgeons, as portrayed on television and in other media, is not a good one. If you have any doubts, just watch one episode of *Nip/Tuck* on the FX cable network. The reason plastic surgeons have such a bad rap is that media coverage usually focuses on consumer vanity and attempts to achieve beautiful bodies in a never-ending search for the Fountain of Youth. But most plastic surgeons aren't like that. And even if they are, what really matters is how good they are at what they do.

It is important that they empathize with your loved one, because what she is undergoing is hard on her emotionally, and it's their job to make her image of herself whole again. So, even though the plastic surgeon doesn't have an impact on her long-term survival chances, he is unbelievably important for rebuilding her self-esteem and self-image. That is, a plastic surgeon's primary job is to make her feel not only like a woman again but also like a complete woman. "When they look at themselves in the mirror, they don't want to be reminded of the loss," according to Dr. Jeffrey A. Ascherman, Chief Plastic Surgeon, Associate Professor of Clinical Surgery, Columbia University Medical Center, who was my wife's plastic surgeon. "Reconstruction helps women put cancer behind them."

· ·

The Medical Army's Code of Conduct for Your Loved One

Once her Medical Army has been assembled, make sure each team member follows the Patient's Bill of Rights, which I like to call the Ten Commandments of Cancer Land:

1. *Quality of Care.* She has the right to the best possible medical treatment available to anyone, anywhere in the world.

2. *Choice*. She has the right to decide the who, what, and where of her treatment, as well as the how and why that treatment is conducted.

3. *Information*. She has the right to be fully educated about her condition, treatment options, and medical qualifications of everyone treating her; the right to examine her records at any time; and the right to fully know and understand what is being done to her at any time during treatment.

4. *Response*. She has the right to a complete and reasonable response to any and all requests she makes of her treating physicians and nurses.

5. *Informed Consent*. She has the right to accept or decline any phase or element of her treatment.

6. *Research*. She has the right to participate in clinical trials if she meets the required criteria.

7. *Continuity*. She has the right to expect the same level of medical care and professionalism if she changes from one doctor to another.

8. *Legal Prerogatives*. She has the right to refuse medical treatment; the right to assign that right to another person under a power of attorney; and the right to complain and appeal any treatment that she feels has wronged her in any way.

9. *Dignity*. She has the right to be respected at all times, in any and all situations.

10. *Privacy*. She has the right to confidentiality with regard to her medical records and communications between and with her doctors.

The Corps

The breast cancer war cannot be won without the Medical Army. Yet it also cannot be fought without the full support and participation of family and friends, fighting alongside her, with you in the trenches each step of the way. These special folks are the friends and family dedicated to her cause of conquering cancer. They are the few, the humble, The Corps.

There is so much more to fighting and beating breast cancer than just the medical battle. That's because the disease attacks the very core of your loved one's femininity. It calls into question all that it means to be a woman—physically, sexually, emotionally, and intellectually. It strategically bombards all relationships she has, and will have, with anyone and everyone in her life, as a wife, girlfriend, significant other, mother, daughter, sister, cousin, friend, coworker. So she is going to need support, a ton of it, to meet all of her emotional and mental needs. To make this work, she is going to need someone who steps up as the leader of her Corps. That person is her chief of staff.

The Chief of Staff

The chief of staff is someone who keeps everything concerning the patient on an even keel. If the patient is married, her chief of staff is usually her husband. But it could just as well be her best friend, her parents, her sister or brother. If she is not married, it could be her boyfriend, parents, or best friend. Whoever it is, that person "must be someone who can run a country," according to breast surgeon Dr. Bob Williams. That's because when someone is diagnosed with breast cancer, it seems like a small country "comes calling." Everyone wants to know everything all at once—how bad her condition is, when she is getting her operation, who her oncologist is, when the lasagna can be dropped off, how the kids are taking it, and of course, there is the ultimate question: how is she doing?

The first assignment for every chief of staff is to get all this chaos under control. The patient is too overwhelmed with her medical decisions to figure out how to handle the social and emotional mayhem. So if you are going to be her chief of staff, the first thing that needs to be done is for you to contain the social tsunami. There are several effective ways to do that, right away.

The very first thing that you can do is to not answer the phone every time it rings. In this age of instant information and constant communication, everyone wants to know everything right away. Well, they can just wait. The key thing for everyone to know is that they will not be told about everything that is happening with her diagnosis and treatment. That's because, in most cases, not everything is known of her true condition until after surgery—at the earliest. So you need to convey to all interested parties, from the start, that they must be respectful of how much the patient wants to reveal to family and friends. She may not want to tell her closest family members, either. That's okay. It is her choice.

As chief of staff, you need to spread out enough information to inform, but not give too much detail. Keep it short, simple, and sweet—and whatever you do, make sure it is always upbeat and positive. The last thing you need to do is create a sense of gloom and doom before treatment has even started. An effective way to get the word out about her treatment is to post updates on websites like caringbridge.org, a not-for-profit organization's website that you can use to link friends and family to your loved one in her time of need. However you spread the word to others, be ready for a cascade of questions (and opinions) about what should and should not be done. That's fine. Just grin, nod, and keep your answers to the bare minimum. Emotions are just too high at this moment; don't let the energy be sucked out of you, your loved one, or anyone else involved by all the know-it-alls, naysayers, and doubting Thomases.

Instead, it's time to circle the wagons and assemble her Corps.

Creating the Corps

"The Corps" is that group of persons who constitute her support team, usually her closest family and friends. Depending on her relationship with others at work, it can also include coworkers and, yes, bosses. Whoever is a member of the Corps must be willing and committed to being her support team. The people in the Corps must be positive, proactive, protective, loving, great listeners, keepers of secrets, and on call, available at a moment's notice. They must also be calming, caring, and concerned. They must know when it is time to step out of the way and when to step into a situation. They need to recognize the time to take orders from her and when not.

The Corps is all about helping. Members will clean the house, take the kids to school, drive her to her doctors' appointments—in short, do everything and anything that needs to be done. They will *always* have her best interests in mind. If she is up for talking, fine, they are there to listen. If she wants time to herself, they don't take it personal.

How does an ex-husband fit into the Corps? Like everyone else, it depends on two things: if she wants him part of the Corps and whether he has the right stuff to manage it. Tim had just separated from his wife, Valerie, when she was diagnosed with breast cancer. He had already been feeling guilty for having left her, and then when she was diagnosed, he felt worse. So Tim resumed his role as husband, taking her to appointments and being there through her surgery. But the sickness didn't fix the marriage; after surgery, his wife wanted him out of her life. He still feels guilty about everything that happened, but he respected her wishes. She wanted to divorce and move on with her life. "We realized that we couldn't be around each other any more," Tim said. "I felt that I was killing her. I felt like a shitty husband." Tim tried to make the marriage work, but it wasn't the best thing for Valerie. The marriage ended.

There are, of course, the toxic ex-husbands who are just no good for her, especially when she's going through breast cancer. With that said, if she shares children with him, there needs to be some understanding, some truce, between them for the best interests of the children. Likewise, if you are the new husband sandwiched between these two people, it's important to stay out of the way and let someone else in the Corps step in to set the ex straight on what he may be doing wrong. Cancer has caused enough chaos already. You don't need to stir up things further.

There's an old saying that friends and family are there for life. It's a good saying, but it doesn't always hold true when your loved one is diagnosed with breast cancer. Many friends and family members simply can't face the prospect of someone they love having a serious disease. Does this mean that they don't love the person? No. What it does mean is that maybe they aren't suited for the Corps.

Sharon had several friends who, when the chips were down, weren't able to be there for her. She had family members drop the ball as well. This, unfortunately, is common when a life-threatening disease rears its ugly head. Why some friends and family can't step up to the cancer challenge is not clear. Maybe they can't deal with their own mortality. Maybe they are scared of "catching" the cancer themselves (even though that is medically impossible). Maybe they don't know how to take care of another human being. Or maybe they are just jerks; if they aren't jerks, maybe they are just acting like jerks right now. The real reason may never be known—and that's okay, because all she needs to know now is who is, and who is not, going to be there for her, through thick and thin.

What is incredibly hard is how to determine who is going to step into the trenches with her and who isn't. There are the people whom you would think could never be any help; there are others whom you can't imagine *not* being anything other than Nurse Florence Nightingale, yet they vanish into the night, never heard from again. Then there is the worst-case scenario in which family and friends say mean, horrible insensitive things and then leave.

One daughter, in her mid-forties, turned to her mom after being diagnosed, desperate for motherly hugs, kisses, and comforts. This mother, however, had an incredible knack for making anything that happened in the world be all about her. Narcissism never had a better friend than this mom. So when the mother first laid eyes on her daughter, who was in the midst of chemo, all she could talk about was how cancer was contagious and had a "smell" about it. Needless to say, she was banished from the daughter's house until after treatment was completed. Toxic people have absolutely no place in the Corps or by your loved one's bedside. Kris Carr, in her book *Crazy Sexy Cancer Tips,* refers to these folks as "emotional vampires that make your cancer all about themselves." But enough talk about the bad apples; let's get back to the Corps. These people are all about her—nothing more and nothing less. They are active, engaged, encouraging, affectionate, supportive; they are into seeing her get better and beating the cancer. They are there to help her get her life back.

Key Corps Officers

The foundation of your loved one's life has been shaken, so the best thing for her to do is reestablish order as quickly as possible. The leader of this effort, the chief of staff, must lead that charge by establishing a positive aura in and around the patient's home. The chief of staff is not alone in this mission but is backed by the following key Corps officers:

Chief Buddy Director (CBD) (aka Best Friend). Your loved one, facing breast cancer, is up against one of the most difficult challenges of her life, so she is going to need one of the most important persons in her life to be there, by her side, each and every step of the way. That is, she is going to need her best friend, or more officially, her chief buddy director. That person could be her college roommate, her neighbor, her childhood friend, her sister, her brother—it doesn't matter. What does matter is that this person be someone whom your loved one is able to call, night or day, to comfort her as she goes through her treatment.

Becky's "best friend" was actually her three sisters. This troika gave Becky a little bit of everything among them. One sister was all about humor; she could make Becky laugh at anything. The second sister was good at talking about serious matters, as well as helping navigate the insurance process. The third sister was her spiritual support, helping tap into a higher power for comfort and consoling.

Chief Dude Director (CDD). This person is your personal chief buddy. That person, whoever it is, is willing to stand by you when *you* are down; it's someone who can drop everything to be by *your* side.

I actually recruited two for my journeys with my wife and sister (whose breast cancers happened one right after the other). The first chief dude was my best friend Bill, who knew me since college and was my roommate when I moved to New York in the mid-1980s. He knew the good, the bad, and the ugly about me, and so he was able to react to anything that I would throw his way. He was also obliging when my wife asked him to get me out of the house because I needed a break. Bill has a dry sense of humor, and he used that to make me laugh in many situations. My second, André, was different from Bill, a sensitive, compassionate, caring man who is also one of the best listeners I have ever known. His day job was as an editor and publisher at a major publishing firm; and I guess his experience with crazy writers was perfect training for handling me, the crazy cancer caregiver.

Chief Fun Officer (CFO). Perhaps the best preparation, mentally, for your loved one embarking on her breast cancer journey is fun. It's also your best preparation as caregiver. There will be plenty of sadness, turmoil, and heartache heading your way, so the last thing she and you need is to be serious all the time. It's time for everyone to rally, and the best way to do that is to throw a party.

When my wife was diagnosed, we organized an F-U Cancer Party. This party was our war cry, an opportunity for friends, family, and coworkers to rally behind Sharon and let her know that she had nothing to fear because she was going to whomp it! To make things extra fun, we hired an Elvis Presley impersonator to serenade Sharon, as she is a huge Elvis fan. Also, if you can't be tacky at a time like this, when can you be? This Elvis, dressed in his Vegas best, was having so much fun that he was one of the last to leave the party. There was a huge cake with candles, for Sharon to make a wish that all would go well with her treatment. Over a hundred people came, many bringing gag gifts. Sharon loved all the attention and the gags, but every person is different. Another friend wanted her F-U Cancer Party to be just her close friends, who brought a variety of pink presents and lots of hugs.

Command, Control, and Communications Officer (CCC). This person is all about operations; he or she must be organized, a taskmaster, committed to making sure everyone signs up and steps up. This person is in charge of organizing all the friends who want to help out but don't know exactly how. The first order of business usually centers on food—who is going to make what dinner when. Nowadays, this is easily done, coordinating dates and dinner deliveries using an Internet or BlackBerry calendar program, but a spiral-bound datebook works as well. Just make sure your loved one isn't served chicken every night! But food coordination is just one of many CCC responsibilities. Another is getting help to do yard work or take care of the dog or drive the children to school. I recommend that this helper access the website lotsahelpinghands.com, useful for creating a virtual community circle.

. . . .

Financial Navy

. . . .

As with any battle, the issue of how a war is to be financed must be addressed and handled properly. Given the high cost of medical treatment today, this is especially important. Her medical bills must be paid in order for her to get her life back in order after treatment. So, the first thing that your loved one should consider, even before selecting her doctors, is to know, in detail, everything about her insurance policy.

The health insurance policy may or may not cover doctors, hospitals, chemotherapy and radiation, clinical trials, nursing care, and home health care. The decisions to be made regarding these are often determined by a patient's financial resources and her extent of insurance coverage. It's no secret that medical expenses are high and getting higher every day. It's vital, then, that your loved one learn the language of medicine and understand the intricacies of her health insurance policy.

If she is an employee, or spouse of an employee at a large corporation, a great place to start is with an Employee Assistance Professional (EAP). It is this person's job to help her navigate the system. Other companies might have what are called medical or nurse advocates. She can always ask for help from someone in the human resources department as well.

If she is an employee of a smaller, or even a medium-size company, such in-house resources are commonly not available, and so she will have to work through the insurance maze herself.

What happens if she doesn't have any health insurance? If she is over the age of sixty-five, she is eligible for coverage under Medicare. If she is indigent, she may be eligible for coverage under Medicaid. There are other federal, state, and private assistance programs she may qualify for as well. To learn more about Medicare, Medicaid, and other federal, state, and private programs, go to http://www.cms .hhs.gov.

Necessary Documentation

Assuming she does have medical insurance, the first step into the insurance morass is to get confirmation, in writing, that all of her doctors and treatment centers (hospitals, cancer centers, etc.) are covered under her policy. If her plan is a preferred provider organization (PPO), then she needs to review the rules for what it means to go in or out of the network of doctors, hospitals, and treatment centers. Doctors bill separately from the place where they provide their services, so she needs to make sure that *both* are covered. Again, to avoid any misunderstanding or denial of coverage, she needs to obtain written preauthorizations from the insurance company before any visit to a specialist or any treatment takes place. With written documentation, she has evidence of being approved for the services she needs, and she won't have to spend hours on the phone later on, trying to get the insurance company to pay the bills.

What happens if the preauthorization for a facility, doctor, or treatment is denied? Well, depending on the insurance policy and the state she lives in, the first step is to appeal that decision. Insurance companies usually must allow patients to appeal their decisions, and often some strong arguments can get the company to reverse its denial of coverage. If not, then the next step is to contact the state's regulatory insurance body to get them to help overturn the decision. It's also not a bad idea to contact elected officials to see what they can do to correct the situation. The louder she protests any inequities, the more likely the insurance company will be interested in settling the claim.

Whatever is discussed with representatives of an insurance company should be confirmed in writing. You want to ensure the fullest medical coverage for your loved one. I'm not saying that all health insurance companies are bad—they aren't. Indeed, for the women in my life, the insurance companies rose to the occasion and covered all claims. But let's not forget that they are in business to make money, so if there are any loopholes, they may try to find them and use them. It's not personal, just business.

The Costs Involved

As more and more companies with comprehensive health plans pass the costs of these plans onto their employees, hospitals and doctors are mining their patients' financial records to determine the likelihood that they will be able to pay their bills; if there is a doubt in their ability to do so, they try to drop them from their patient rolls. The *Wall Street Journal* reported that Experian, the huge credit-reporting company, bought SearchAmerica, of Maple Grove, Minnesota, a company that specializes in analyzing patient incomes and payment capabilities. SearchAmerica creates a patient "healthcare credit score," similar to the FICO scores for credit purposes, and examines whether patients are eligible for federal, state, or local assistance in addition to any insurance coverage they may have. The big question is this: as hospitals increasingly turn to establishing creditworthiness as a standard for care, will that translate to more breast cancer patients being denied the treatment they need?

It is always important for your loved one to never have a gap in insurance coverage, if she can help it. Since she has been diagnosed with breast cancer, she will always have the mark of a "preexisting condition" on any insurance she seeks in the future. The best way to ensure continued coverage is to never miss a premium payment. If she is between jobs, she can keep her previous coverage by paying for it through the COBRA program, which stands for the Consolidated Omnibus Budget Reconciliation Act. COBRA gives her the same coverage that she had before—for a price, of course, which is what the company paid for her coverage when she was employed. Coverage under COBRA extends anywhere from eighteen to twenty-six months after she leaves her company, depending on her circumstances.

When your loved one is putting together her financial strategy, she should know that not all doctors, or facilities, bill equally. It is a good idea to ask what things cost, before incurring those charges. I recently learned that scans ordered by my wife's oncologist from a particular hospital cost triple what they would have cost at a third-party imaging center for the exact same quality of service. She went to the imaging center.

However broad your loved one's insurance coverage is, there will be a flurry of bills coming in. So, it's important to start getting all those medical bills and insurance forms in order. Someone should set up a folder system to organize and track the bills received and the benefits approved and paid for by her insurance company. There are several software programs available to help with this—Quicken Medical Expense Manager being one of them.

• • •

What if she can't pay the bills, for whatever reason? It would be a mistake to forgo treatment, yet that's what people in dire straits sometimes do. You don't want your loved one to be among them. If there's no health insurance, and she doesn't qualify for aid, an alternative could be to take out a home equity line on the house or condo, assuming of course there is equity in it. This option should be one of last resort, however, since she could lose her house or condo if she doesn't pay back the home equity loan in a timely manner.

Perhaps a better solution for her might be to declare bankruptcy so she can settle the debts at a lower interest rate and/or adjusted principal. If she charged her doctors' payments, treatments, medications, etc., to her credit card, she could later negotiate with the medical providers, as well as with the credit card companies, to lower the interest rate or stretch out the payments; the downside of this is that her credit history would be harmed.

. . . .

Soul Air Force

. . . .

To beat cancer, your loved one must have the *will* to win, which for some women has to come from on high or within themselves. My sister Mary, a devout Catholic, credits faith for getting her through her personal breast cancer battle. "It was God's inspiration that let me know I would be prepared," she says. "He gets all the credit."

Whether she is religious or not, she may feel that there is some "other" voice, or some "higher power," that gives her spiritual guidance and comfort, and on which she relies to determine the right thing to do, commonly referred to as her "inner voice."

Whether that voice comes to her from God, herself, or John Lennon, it doesn't matter. Yep, that's right—whatever works for her. For my mom, she prayed to St. John Neumann, a saint whose claim to fame was that he was one of the first bishops to establish the Roman Catholic schools in the United States. His shrine was about a half hour from my mom's house, in Philadelphia. She would make regular visits to St. John with my sister, Mary, and her best friend, Caryl. Mom liked Neumann because he was close to her house and she could talk directly to him, since his body could be seen encased in glass under the altar of the shrine. My sister, also religious, turned to the Virgin Mary to heal her cancer. She traveled overseas to sites where the Virgin Mary has been seen.

My wife turned to Reiki for her spiritual healing. She would visit her Reiki master several times a month in Neptune, New Jersey, on the Jersey Shore. During her chemo treatments, when she wasn't feeling up for driving, I would drop her off for her one-hour session. Her teacher, Karla LaVoie, lived in a nondescript ranch house in a suburban development. I remember a cluster of bright pink plastic flamingos and a plastic palm tree in the yard, and thinking how great it would be in Florida, drinking piña coladas with my wife instead of watching her ingest toxic cancer cocktails.

When Karla went around the room asking each person why he or she was there, most said they wanted to learn new ways to heal their patients, as they were nurses and massage therapists. According to Sharon, "I said I felt that I needed to heal myself. It was sort of embarrassing, but I really did feel that. And every time I would do Reiki on myself, my hand would naturally go to my chest. The training was the most powerful spiritual experience I had or have ever had—it was life altering. I used the Reiki as a relaxation technique and would do it on myself often when lying on medical tables, getting blood drawn, or getting chemo. I also used it when I was stressed out, had insomnia, or just in need of a little peace."

The thing that I remember most about Reiki, and how it worked for my wife, was how intensely she concentrated to create energy and heat for her body. Reiki was all about the placement of Sharon's hands on her infected breast, to make it not only feel better but be better, through healing. "Reiki is a hands-on healing modality that helps to put the patient in a much more relaxed state so that healing can happen from within," according to Sharon's teacher Karla.

Karla explained, "The thing that I do remember about Sharon is her amazingly positive attitude. She was white-hot passionate about becoming healed. When working with people experiencing severe illness, I often help them to imagine a warrior, an inner symbol that will help them fight the cancer. This process is used to complement the medical intervention being done, such as chemotherapy or radiation. Some clients have imagined wolves destroying the cancer inside. Some have seen firemen with hoses, hosing down the cancer so that it is completely released. A couple of people have seen Joan of Arc, St. Michael, or soldiers. Some will imagine that there is a divine laser beam of light that destroys, clears, and releases.

"One woman actually had a very powerful plant growing inside her. It would go to where the cancer was and squeeze it until the cancer was completely annihilated. At the same time the leaves of the plant would surround, bless, and protect her organs."

Religion and Reiki are just two weapons available to your loved one for her spiritual army. Others include meditation, aromatherapy, visualization therapy, massage, yoga, Pilates, herbs, steam baths, hot rocks, and acupuncture. Whatever her approach, the goal is always the same: finding and establishing a purpose that will provide her with internal powers to overcome breast cancer.

The Battle Begins

Surgery

....

MY WIFE LOOKED UP at me with tears in her eyes as she handed me her wedding ring before she was wheeled into the operating room for her mastectomy. Lying there on that gurney, in her surgical gown and covered with a lightweight white blanket, she was living the most vulnerable moment of her life. What was going to happen to us as a married couple after surgery? she thought. What if I didn't want her anymore? Would I always view her as damaged goods? I leaned over, kissed her, and assured her that she had absolutely nothing to worry about. I had no way of knowing that, of course. I gave Sharon one last hug, and then, just like that, she was gone.

As I watched the doors flap back and forth where she had just passed through, I could only imagine the fear and worry that my dad faced when he watched my mom taken away for her operation, back in 1978. That was a time before annual mammograms, before sonograms, MRIs, and PET scans. That was a time when my mom went into surgery not knowing if she had breast cancer or not. It was when a signed consent form gave the surgeon, not her, the decision to remove her breast if cancer was found. My mom didn't know until she woke up in the recovery room if she had breast cancer, and even worse, if she still had her breast or not. When breast cancer was found back then, the surgical attack was aggressive—usually a radical mastectomy, whereby the surgeon removed not only breast tissue but the pectoralis major and pectoralis minor chest muscles, as well as all axillary lymph nodes up to her collarbone. That's how my mom was treated. She learned that she had lost her breast when her friend Caryl took my mom's hand to touch the empty space where her breast once was.

Twenty-three years later, it was my wife's turn to face the loss of her breast; only this time, it would be her decision, not the surgeon's. And it wasn't an easy one to make. When she found out that she had breast cancer, Sharon was instantly committed to saving her breast, and she made a promise to herself to do everything in her power to save it. Early in the process, it seemed that this was the right decision for her. She had one lump, it was small, and medical studies had shown that, given her diagnosis, she had the same long-term survival rates with a lumpectomy as with entire breast removal.

"I went 'animal' on the research into surgical procedures," according to Sharon. "Information was my only sense of control, so I pushed my intellect to its capacity, taking on the medical knowledge and weighing everything as rationally as possible, while still allowing my gut instinct to guide me in the end." Given her diagnosis, all roads seemed to lead her to a lumpectomy—until Dr. Marc Brown, a radiologist at Columbia University in New York City, found a second lump on the edge of Sharon's films that the first radiologist had missed. After the second tumor proved cancerous, Sharon was left with no other choice than to get a mastectomy—and face her deep-seated fear that, by losing her breasts, she would be losing her femininity, her sexuality, her maternity, her inner "her."

. . . .

Getting Ready for Battle

. . . .

If your loved one has been diagnosed with breast cancer, she will almost always be treated surgically, first with an initial biopsy and then later with a lumpectomy, mastectomy, or bilateral mastectomy. Additional surgery may be done on her lymph nodes. A mastectomy is usually followed with reconstructive surgery by a plastic surgeon, right after the breast surgeon has completed his or her work in the same operating room.

Emotional scars often follow the physical scars created by breast surgery. In one of the earliest research studies on the psychological impact of breast cancer surgery on women, cited by Dr. Barron Lerner in his book *Breast Cancer Wars*, Richard Renneker, a psychiatrist, and Max Cutler, a breast surgeon, concluded that a woman's breast is "the emotional symbol of a woman's pride in her sexuality and her motherhood," so that a removal of her breast attacked the "very core" of her "feminine orientation."

Breast cancer surgery is an invasion of a woman's natural body. It's every woman's nightmare. Women, just like men, want to be considered physically and sexually attractive, and breasts play a large part in that attractiveness. To say that body image is important to women is an understatement. Everywhere we look today there are images of the "ideal," the "perfect" woman. Who is this woman? She works, she works out, she manages the house, she's a sex kitten, she never complains, she's organized, she's intelligent, and on top of all that, she is a knockout. We see her everywhere—on magazine covers, on television shows, in movies, on billboards and CD covers.

It takes a lot of courage, then, for a woman to face breast surgery. That's why this chapter is the color purple. The Purple Heart, awarded by the U.S. military, is given to those select few men and women who have been wounded or killed in battle, and who have given their blood defending their homeland. They "shall forever be revered" by their countrymen, according to a military edict issued by George Washington as commander-in-chief of the Continental Army in 1782. Purple symbolizes royalty—those of the highest rank—because in ancient times purple cloth was the rarest of colors, making it the symbol of kings and queens.

Breast surgery is a royal rite of passage into Cancer Land. It's a journey filled with monsters, dangerous cliffs, and seemingly impossible obstacles. Every journey through Cancer Land is unique, challenging, and full of the unknown. What is known is that it will teach her, and you, how precious and important life is. So get ready—the ultimate battle with cancer is set to begin.

The Breast Surgeon

The first element of any surgery is its scheduling. The better the surgeon, the longer the wait, so as mentioned in the previous chapter, the sooner she gets on the surgeon's calendar, the better. The surgery is usually scheduled after the initial consultation with the surgeon, when the doctor goes over everything that is going to happen before, during, and after surgery. The initial consultation is a detailed review of what the surgeon plans to do to get the cancer out of her body. It's the surgeon's battle plan. Often, this initial consultation is the first time the patient, and her loved ones, realize that the breast cancer is for real and not just a bad dream.

During this consultation, the surgeon should discuss everything that he or she plans to do with her breast or breasts. That is, the surgeon should review where exactly the incision is going to be made, how much of the breast or breasts the surgeon plans to remove, and any and all possible complications that could occur. Medical information can get lost in translation from surgeon to patient, so Dr. Roxanne Davenport, a Virginia breast surgeon, strongly urges that a patient have a loved one in the room with her to be her active listener. If it is a husband, and the wife wants him to weigh in on a decision, then he should do it right then, in the room, Davenport says. Just saying that he supports whatever she wants to do is not enough. He needs to be on the record as being behind what is going to be done, as decided by his wife.

The surgical consultation is *the* time to ask any questions of the doctor so that there are no surprises later. She, and you as her caregiver, need to know everything about what to expect. Be sure the surgeon answers all of her questions. Ideally, she will have all her questions written down beforehand, in order of priority. She and her active listener should take copious notes. And don't be afraid to get clarifications on the answers that are given. That initial consultation should take forty-five minutes to an hour; ask for more time if she can get it, too. Also, she, and you, should leave open the possibility for follow-up questions, by e-mail, phone, or another office visit—whichever works best to get the best answers from the surgeon.

The most important thing to come out of that initial meeting is trust—trust between the patient and doctor, not between the doctor and you. "I always felt that I had to be comfortable and confident with my patients before operating on them," remarked my wife's breast cancer surgeon, Dr. Beth Ann Ditkoff. "There is a two-way trust element between patient and surgeon that cannot be underestimated."

So how can she, and you, trust her surgeon? It's true that you can't always tell who people really are from first impressions, but with surgeons you can, and here's why: surgeons are extremely busy folks, and they don't have time to put on airs or assume other personalities. So after all the consultations, screenings, reviews, and discussions, if her gut says to go with a particular surgeon, then that's it.

The Anesthesiologist

The second doctor to consider in the operating room is the anesthesiologist. Putting someone to sleep and bringing that person back safely is an exact and complicated science. So having your loved one find out who is taking care of this part of the operation, and how that person is going to do it, is a vital item on her medical checklist.

There are a number of things to learn about the anesthesiologist. Start with the person's experience, such as how many breast cancer procedures he or she has been involved with. Learn about what drugs the doctor plans to apply and why, the dosage to be given, and the risks involved. Ask who will be monitoring her vital signs during the operation and how that is done. What effect, if any, will the drug or drugs have on her vital signs—heart rate, blood pressure, oxygen saturation levels? How long will she be "under," and how long will the recovery phase take? How long has the anesthesiologist worked with this team, and what is the team's experience with breast cancer? What are the side effects expected in the recovery room? Is there anything she can do beforehand (e.g., things she should or shouldn't eat or drink) to minimize bad side effects? It's important for her to tell the anesthesiologist if she has had any bad reactions in the past to drugs, either in the operating room, or with medications, as well as provide information about any allergic reactions. She should know what the doctor will do if there is a harsh reaction to the administered drugs or, worse, if critical functions are compromised. What emergency procedures are in place, and how often have these been applied? Don't be afraid to ask if the doctor has had direct experience in such a situation. Does her anesthesiologist know how to use resuscitation or life-support equipment?

There is no reason to be short on questions at this, or any other, stage of the surgical process. Knowledge is power and offers greater assurance of success.

The Plastic Surgeon

If a plastic surgeon is going to be involved with reconstruction right after the breast surgery, then there should be an initial consultation with that doctor as well. With reconstructive surgery, it is important to know the relationship the plastic surgeon has with the breast surgeon and their past experience in working together. Your loved one should feel as comfortable with the plastic surgeon as she does with her breast surgeon. During her consultation, a discussion should ensue that reviews how the transference will occur in the operating room between the breast surgeon and plastic surgeon. Also, she should ask what complications could occur with reconstruction. Lastly, she should request to see past work done by the plastic surgeon, and ask to talk to some of his patients who went through the same procedure to hear their perspectives.

The Location

Where the operation will take place may be as important as the doctors selected. The equipment, operating room, operating procedures, nursing staff, and support staff all affect the outcome of breast cancer surgery. The more experience the hospital staff has in treating breast cancer, the better the chances of her recovery from the surgery—and for the rest of her life.

It seems, at first, that a big selling point for any hospital is its proximity to the patient's home. This is always a plus, but if she has complications with her diagnosis, a Comprehensive Cancer Center or university hospital may be a better option for her surgery. To help decide which is best, contact the hospitals involved and ask for the quality office, then ask how many breast cancer operations are done at that hospital, as well as its success and complication rates with this type of surgery.

The Insurance

After the surgical team and hospital are secured, the mundane—yet crucial—pieces of the process need to come together, and this includes preauthorization. That's right. She must be darn sure that the doctors and hospital (never assume the doctors and hospital are together) she has selected are approved for coverage (or in the network) under her health plan. Usually the doctor's office staff are well versed in this and equipped to get the paperwork together for the insurance company. The burden to do so, however, is not on them, but on her, so make sure she fills out all the forms needed to get the operation into the insurer's system. Failure to do so could result in delay, or even cancellation, of the surgery. Or, the surgery could go forward, and the insurance company might then refuse to pay the bills because the medical procedures were not authorized. The latter, indeed, could prove to be a financial disaster. More people go bankrupt owing to an inability to pay medical bills than for any other reason, including mortgage foreclosures, car loans, and credit card debt.

. . . .

The Final Prep Checklist

. . . .

The final prep is all about getting her ready for her operation. She'll pack most of the things that she'll need herself, but it's not a bad idea to help her get ready and to bring along a few things that could surprise her and cheer her up, like the following.

Music. My wife loves her tunes. It is incredible how music soothes her in times of trouble. When she went to the hospital back in 2001, it was before the omnipresence of iPods, so I brought along a boom box that played a CD mix of her favorite songs, which she could listen to to calm her nerves before and after surgery. If you are into music, and you know the kind of music that will make your loved one relax, make her a music mix as a special gift to her.

Photographs/Sculptures/Scripture/Poetry. Another great thing to bring along to the hospital are photographs—of loved ones, special places, or other things that give her inspiration and strength. A friend of a stem cell transplant patient, who wasn't allowed real flowers in the room because of the risk of infection, took a photograph of a different flower each day, printed it out, and posted that photo on the patient's wall each morning. The patient was going to be in the hospital for weeks, yet within days the hospital walls were transformed into a spectacular flower garden. Every day the patient couldn't wait to find out what the new flower of the day would be.

Bring along, then, whatever will bring her joy and inspiration during her hospital stay. It could be a small sculpture, a quotation from her favorite writer or scripture, her favorite scented candle, drawings from her children, or a poem. When Sharon went to the hospital, I got our young boys to draw pictures and write notes to their mommy about how much they loved her and how proud they were of her fighting cancer. This encouragement from my children continues to this day. Recently, I was looking through Barack Obama's *Dreams of my Father*, which my oldest son Seth gave Sharon for Mother's Day. On the first page, he wrote, "I could have never asked for a better mother. You are a survivor not only of Isaac and me, but also of a terrible disease. There are not many women who can go through chemo without even 'acting phased' in front of her kids. You rock. Love, Seth. *XOXO*."

Visitor VIPs. Who comes to visit your loved one in the hospital is entirely up to her. Every woman has a different list, and each one is the *final* list. Your job, if you are the primary caregiver, is to be the bouncer, allowing only those from her select VIP list entry and moving visitors out of her room when they overstay their welcome. Usually, immediate family is invited, but not always. Sharon initially had only three people on her visitation list—myself, her brother David, and Caryl, my mom's best friend and herself a breast cancer survivor. One of the reasons she picked us three is that none of us had "real" breasts. After surgery, when she felt a bit better, she wanted to have her boys with her, as well as one of her best friends from when she was growing up. No more, no less. It was what worked for her.

My sister Mary's invite list included her husband, Joe, Joe's sister, and my wife. She didn't feel comfortable having her three boys, whom she felt were too young at the time, visit a hospital; she didn't want them to see the anguish she was going through by having to face the same disease that killed our mom fourteen years before. My mom had the shortest guest list of all. She had only her best friend, Caryl, beside her and my dad. No kids were allowed or any other friends or family until she was almost fully recovered.

Some women want everyone to come and say hi; others will want no one there. As far as the latter, I encourage women to have at least one visitor, because no one should suffer breast cancer surgery alone. Human touch and affection go a long way toward a healthful recovery.

················

Preparing the Home

················

Her doctors will handle what happens at the hospital. But what happens when she comes home? Someone needs to help her prepare, in advance, for everything to be ready for that return from the hospital. First and foremost, there will need to be a person, or persons, at the hospital when she is discharged. Talk over with her who will bring her home.

Next, there has to be someone, or a couple of people, to be with her at home when she arrives. Full recovery from breast surgery can range from two to six weeks, or more. In the beginning, she is not going to do, or want to do, anything for anyone, including herself. So she is going to need help—a lot of help. Her insurance policy may provide for home health care during the first few days or weeks, but if not, she is going to need volunteers to take care of her.

If she has kids living at home, how and what happens to them is also an important part of the home considerations. Sit with her, then, before she goes to the hospital to figure out her children's schedules: how and when they get up, go to school, get picked up, come and go for sports and music lessons, and so on. And that's just the beginning. There is the food plan: when family members eat, what they eat, even how they eat.

It is good to have someone in charge of the meals, not only those cooked by someone at home but also those being delivered by concerned family and friends. This is a great project to give to visiting parents. This is what I did with my mother-in-law Mary Rapoport, who is probably the most competent person ever in the kitchen. Martha Stewart's got nothing on her. Her day job is to promote eggs for the Virginia Egg Council, and she is a major force at the annual White House Easter Egg Roll. So she had her list of meals and her deliveries run as if it was being put on by the White House, perhaps even better. The meals were coordinated and varied, so we never had lasagna or chicken casserole two nights in a row. I never ate so well in my life, thanks to her.

Then there is getting the physical house in order. If your loved one is fortunate enough to have a cleaning service, they can continue to keep the house presentable. If not, then you as caregiver will have to recruit one or more persons who will regularly, and not in a disruptive way, keep the floors clean, dishes done, clothes washed, and everything else in order. If your loved one is like most women, she wants her house presentable for guests when they come to visit her after surgery.

As if that weren't enough, there is the need to convert her bedroom into the "comfort zone." Your loved one will be going through major surgery, so she will need to have her bed stocked with comfy pillows and blankets. She will need easy access to her bathroom. She will also need pain medications and anti-infection medications. Someone needs to go to the local pharmacy to get these drugs *before* she gets home, if she isn't released with a carryover supply of medication. The refrigerator should also be stocked with food and drink that won't upset her stomach. Most important, you need to make sure that, in the comfort zone, she will be able to get uninterrupted sleep, rest, and relaxation. Your loved one is going to be bombarded with well-meaning family members, friends, and coworkers who will want to stop by, or call, to see just how she is doing. Someone will need to coordinate this onslaught, a gatekeeper who can schedule visits and then change them based on how she is feeling. To keep folks from just dropping in, post a note on the door saying your loved one is resting, and thanks for stopping by. You can also leave a pen and paper outside the door so they can write a note of support. Consider taking the phone out of her room (with her permission, of course), so it doesn't ring and wake her when she's sleeping.

. . . .

The Night Before Surgery

. . . .

Leading up to the surgery, there may be an irrational hope from your loved one that somehow the diagnosis is wrong, that somehow the films were switched, that the cancer shown on those films is in someone else's body. It's easy to see how this feeling can arise. After all, there appears to be nothing physically wrong with her! There is no outward appearance of cancer. Surgery, however, changes cancer from concept to harsh reality. So the night before surgery, for most cancer patients (and for their loved ones, too) is often when all her pent-up anxieties, anticipations, worries, and fears scare the bejesus out of her—and you. Because the full extent of her cancer cannot be known until after surgery and the pathology is completed, it's easy to imagine that the worst is yet to come.

The most important thing that needs to happen the night before surgery is that she follow her surgeon's pre-op orders, which often include not eating after midnight, getting plenty of rest, and drinking only clear fluids (preferably just water).

....

The Day of Battle: Healing with Steel

....

This is the time for her to put on her game face. For Sharon, that meant being a warrior. She wasn't going to lose to this cancer; she was going to whip it. She needed to "zone in" and get ready for her quest to conquer cancer. I needed to put my game face on, too, as her biggest fan and supporter.

Get her to the hospital on time. There is a lot of medical preparation that happens right before surgery, so don't be late. There is also emotional preparation. For your loved one, that emotional prep is accepting that she is facing, head-on, a radical change in her life. As Sharon put on her surgical gown and laid down on the gurney to be wheeled into the operating room, she was overwhelmed with sadness that she was about to lose a part of herself. "I had always loved my breasts," she said. "I felt they were perfect. A lot of women wish their breasts were bigger or smaller, but I always liked mine. The saddest part of all, for some weird reason, was giving up that part of me that had suckled my boys. Breast-feeding was one of the most fulfilling things I ever experienced, and I didn't want to lose the part of my body that had made that possible for me. It was like losing a really close, much beloved friend. It was terribly, terribly sad." Right behind that sadness loomed a tower of fear that Sharon admitted to me only afterwards: "I wasn't sure how you would feel toward me as a woman. I was afraid I would gross you out and you'd try to hide it, but I'd know and that would kill me."

The best thing that a caregiver can do on the day of her surgery is to be there for her, listening and supporting her. But you also need to work with her medical team, the group she chose to save her life. So do what they ask you to do, for her. It is hard to turn your loved one over to strangers, but they have her best interests in mind. Trust them as she does. There's nothing more that you can do for her at this point but believe that all will go well. It's okay to be afraid of what is going to happen next. Just keep that worry to yourself.

Then it's time for her to leave you. It is at that moment that you both realize that everything after that moment will change, forever. It's time to say good-bye to that past—together—and immediately turn to the new, challenging future, which begins in the operating room where the doctors begin their magic. If your loved one is having a lumpectomy, the procedure is usually less than an hour. If she is having a mastectomy, then the procedure can last an hour or more. And if there is immediate reconstruction done right after that, then her surgical time will be even longer.

In addition to the removal of the tumor or tumors, there must be an exploration beyond the site to see if the cancer has spread. The first place doctors look is in the axillary lymph nodes. It is standard procedure to test if the axillary nodes have been infected by cancerous cells, and they do this by conducting a sentinel node biopsy. This involves injection of either a dye or a radioactive agent that indicates whether the sentinel, or first node, has been infected. If cancer is found there, then more nodes are tested, and if found positive, are removed.

The hardest part for any caregiver during surgery is the wait. You can't see what is happening in there, and so you just wander around the waiting room, picking through outdated magazines, watching bad reality TV on a screen five times too small for the room, and drink burnt coffee with fake creamer—until her surgeon comes into the room with the news about the operation. Some surgeons recommend that family members go home and come back at a certain time; I don't advocate this, if for no other reason than I think it is reassuring to your loved one, and you, that you are there for her, literally, until she is in the clear. It's not that doing so makes the operation go better, or faster; but it does give her, I think, more comfort than if no one were out there, watching out for her. Unfortunately, some women go to their surgery with no companion, perhaps because they are single or divorced, or have no friends or family members in town. This has to be the loneliest feeling in the world.

When the surgeon does finally come out of the operating room to the waiting room, you don't want to miss him or her, because the doctor won't come back. The surgeon will tell you how the operation went, but to get more information than that you have to be the person whose name your loved one gave written permission on the appropriate consent form to receive her surgery details. Medical information is considered private, protected under the Health Insurance Portability and Accountability Act, or HIPAA. But assuming you are named on the release, have your list of questions ready for the surgeon. Ask whether she had any complications, if she had any positive lymph nodes, or nodes the doctor is concerned about. Ask if the transfer to the plastic surgeon went well, and how long the doctor thinks it will be before the pathology comes back from the lab.

Some women have chemotherapy treatments before surgery. This usually is the route if the tumor or tumors in the breast are quite large. The doctors want to shrink the tumors before surgery and the chemo can do that. Some breast cancer treatment centers give chemotherapy to patients before surgery, no matter what size her tumors are. M.D. Anderson Cancer Center in Houston, Texas, for example, has made chemo a standard presurgery procedure for tumors 2 centimeters or larger. The reasoning is that, if the tumor shrinks enough, then that reduces the chances of the patient's having to lose her breast, instead opting for a lumpectomy. The upside of this approach is that, in some instances, the tumors not only shrink but may disappear altogether. The other advantage is that oncologists can observe what chemo drugs are working and what aren't, based on how the tumors react. But there is a downside to this approach as well. The cancer's presence in the lymph nodes may be eliminated, which then removes a risk indicator for effectively determining the chances of a recurrence.

......

The Plastic Surgery

......

If she is having plastic surgery done as part of her breast cancer surgery operation, a second consultation in that waiting room will occur with the plastic surgeon when he or she is finished. Again, ask if there were any complications, how the doctor felt the operation went, and details on what to expect in the coming days, as well as what needs to be done for her at home.

A lot of thought goes into the reconstruction of a breast or breasts before that surgery is done. The first is what type of operation she wants to have. Most women opt for implants, which are sacs filled with either saline or silicon. With implants, the first procedure is usually to insert a tissue expander under the chest muscle and to expand it with saline at regular intervals. This stretches the skin so that an implant can be properly placed. Sharon opted for the breast implants, in no small part because our two boys at home were just seven and five years old, so she wanted the quickest recovery. Before the surgery, Sharon's plastic surgeon had made surgical marks on her breasts to guide him during the procedure. This marking sort of unnerved her because she wasn't ready for it. "That really weirded me out—it made me feel like an inanimate object," she said. Betsy, in her mid-forties, likewise wasn't advised of this before by her doctor, and she had planned to wear a dress with a plunging neckline to a gala ball right before the operation; but they marked her so much that she thought she resembled a checkerboard, so she opted for a different dress.

Whatever implant or implants are chosen, a woman who has had a mastectomy often may lose sensation in part or all of her breast area, which can leave her feeling that this part of her body, in some ways, no longer exists. This becomes an even bigger problem in the bedroom if the wife and husband's sexual intimacy involved stimulation of her breasts during foreplay and intercourse. It's important to note that some skilled oncoplastic surgeons are now performing skin sparing and nipple sparing procedures, when appropriate, to salvage some, or all, of the breast sensations.

If your loved one is going to have radiation later, there needs to be a discussion between the plastic surgeon and the radiation oncologist about the impact radiation will have on her implants. For some patients, doctors advise them to get their implants done first, before radiation, since the radiation can shrink and tighten the outer tissue, making it difficult to use the breast expander later. The worst-case scenario is an inability to insert an implant, resulting in a patient's having to use a prosthetic breast made of foam or silicone, depending on how real, and comfortable, she wants it to be.

There are, of course, women who choose to forgo reconstructive surgery. If that is your loved one's decision, you must accept it as final and not fight it. My mom chose this route. Back in the 1970s, when she was diagnosed, she was given fewer than six months to live, and so she didn't see the need to go through the hassle of reconstructive surgery. Nonetheless, she refused to accept their prognosis and underwent an experimental regimen of chemotherapy, which saved her life. Several years later, she still had not gotten reconstructive surgery because, according to her, she was so used to her prosthetic that she gave her "yellow clothed boob" a name: Matilda.

Still other women opt for more extensive surgery by having what is called a TRAM flap procedure, which moves the tranverse rectus abdomini myocutaneous muscle (a major muscle in the stomach), with the fat and skin, to make a breast. The benefit for women is that they have a real flesh-and-blood breast that feels natural and, in the process, get a tummy tuck to boot. Another reconstruction option for a woman is the LAT flap procedure, which takes muscle from the latissimus dorsi in the back. The thought in both of these procedures is that the implant is part of her natural body.

There are several other, new reconstruction techniques. One is called the gluteal flap construction, whereby the surgeon removes skin from the woman's buttocks and grafts it to her breast. There is also the DIEP flap (deep inferior epigastric perforator), which takes fat and skin from the lower abdomen. Just like the TRAM flap, it is a "free flap," taking the muscle to supply blood to the flap, with the blood vessels from the muscle being reattached at the new site. All of these surgical procedures are more intensive procedures and require longer times for the patient to fully recover.

Whichever reconstruction approach she chooses, usually the work is done at the same time as when the cancer is removed from her breast. If there is a second reconstruction operation after surgery, chemotherapy, and/or radiation, the fears and feelings of that first operation might come roaring back; it really depends on the woman.

You should never inject your personal agenda, such as mentioning how you would like her breasts to look—larger, smaller, perkier, enlarged nipples, whatever. I should know. I made that tragic mistake, sitting in the plastic surgeon's examination office as he was taking measurements for the upcoming operation. I wanted to know what the options were for her to, maybe, uh, go up a cup size. Well, I got a blank stare from the plastic surgeon, and I saw the gates of hell in my wife's eyes. To take possession of her body at any time is never good, but it is really bad when she is in such a vulnerable state.

She may want to change her breasts to make them different from before—and that's fine, too. Whatever works for her, not you. After all, it is her self-image that has been compromised here, and it is that self-image that needs to be made whole again—thanks to the magical work of plastic surgeons. Physical reconstruction is just the beginning of many steps she will take to a complete reconstruction of her life. How she feels about her physical self goes a long way toward how she feels about you, her family, her work, and the rest of the world.

····················
Post-op
····················

When Sharon woke up from her operation, the first person she saw was a nurse. The first thing she felt was extreme nausea, so she started puking. The nurse touched Sharon on the shoulder, rubbed her back as she vomited into a bedpan, and said, "I've been where you are. I am a survivor, too." The sisterhood bond had formed right then. "My nurse became my guardian angel. She said that she had been right where I was now, and that I was going to be fine. I felt such love coming from her and I loved her right back. What a gift."

The next gift that she wanted was me—her husband—to embrace her with unconditional love. Pay close attention to what I am about to tell you. This next paragraph is worth the price of admission, not only for this book but possibly for the future happiness of your marriage if she is your wife. Got your attention?

When you first lay eyes on your wife, after surgery, you must not only show your love, but say so, truthfully and with utter sincerity. This is the moment to show her that you are going to Stand by Her—no matter what. If you say or do anything that is not completely honest, it will be a long time before you earn her trust again. When you see her for the first time, after her breast surgery, this is the most vulnerable moment in her life, so don't blow it. Oh, and one other tip: don't say that you like her new breasts better. Bad idea. Really bad.

When I first saw Sharon after surgery, and she looked up at me with those beautiful brown eyes flecked with green, her body shook from the aftereffects of the anesthesia drugs. She wanted to show me, right then, the scar from her operation. She wanted me to accept her, there and then, for who she was. And she wanted to know how I would react to what I saw. So she lifted up her gown and showed me her reconstructed breast.

I looked, and then I touched the side of her face, tears pouring down my cheeks. I looked into her eyes and said, "You are more beautiful to me now than ever before." And it was true. She never looked prettier to me than at that moment. She was perfect, in all ways. It was then that Sharon started to cry as well—tears of relief that everything was going to be fine between us.

A lot can happen during surgery, and a lot can happen in post-surgery. Many patients, like Sharon, suffer nausea. Other complications include bleeding and infections, but these risks are usually not severe and are treated effectively right away. Fluids also collect, which pool in what are referred to as seromas, which are drained into a plastic bag that your loved one will carry around with her for the first few days after surgery.

Another major complication that can result from surgery is lymphedema, or arm swelling, which happens when lymph nodes are removed. This condition can be mild or severe, varying from swollen fingers to an entire swollen arm, sometimes two or more times its normal size. When the lymph nodes are removed, the body no longer can effectively process all the bacteria and other foreign substances, like scar tissue, from the breast operation. Think of the lymphatic system as an internal plumbing system; with lymphedema, that system has broken down. Luckily, lymphedema can be prevented with exercises after surgery and by wearing a compression band around the arm. It is also a good idea to elevate the arm to lower any swelling. There are special arm sleeves that can reduce swelling as well. Sentinel node biopsies have helped to lower axillary surgery by first testing to see if the sentinal node is positive with cancer before proceeding further.

When your loved one finally gets to her hospital bed, the number one priority should be to get her as comfortable as possible.

This begins with pain medications. If she is in pain when she gets to her room, don't be bashful to head to the nurse's station to make them aware that she needs more pain meds. The drug of choice after surgery is morphine. Your loved one will be handed a button that she can push whenever the first inkling of discomfort comes her way. Don't worry. There are a limited number of morphine hits that the machine allows each hour, so she won't overdose. With that said, if she is in pain, and especially if she is trying to be all Rambo about not needing the meds while squirming in agony, do everything in your power to get her to push that button. The best thing she can do for herself, right then, is to rest her body so she can recover.

The hospital staff often will place pneumatic sleeves on her legs that expand and contract to prevent blood clots from forming. She may develop rashes or swellings as a result of the surgery, which will cause discomfort. Again, speak with the staff to have these conditions treated, so she is comfortable at all times.

If you are a husband or boyfriend, remember to convey to your loved one after surgery that she is your warrior-goddess, prettier and better than ever. She needs to hear you say that you love her. You need to be as verbal, sincere, and emotional as you can. She is looking to you for validation that you are still attracted to her. You need her to feel that you are truly there for her. This can be strongly conveyed nonverbally through a touch, hug, kiss, or stroke of her hair. It is so important for the guy not only to be there, but also to touch. Show her you love her just as much as you tell her.

She may want to show you the surgery scar under her gown, and she may not. Let her do what she feels most comfortable doing. If she does show you, as mentioned earlier, this is a hugely vulnerable moment for her. When she lifts that gown, she is most likely not going to be looking at the scar and bandages, but your face and how you react. If ever there were a test of love and support, this is it. You cannot, under any circumstances, show any reaction of concern or, God forbid, disgust. If you are the squeamish type, tell her that and she should understand. The key here is that she not only knows, but also feels, your love at this critical time.

. . . .

The Pathology Report

. . . .

Depending on the extent of the surgery, your loved one could be in the hospital from a day to up to a week—or more, if there are complications. Meantime, the doctors are working to determine what type of cancer she has and exactly where it is located. Pathology sets the stage for everything that happens after this: chemotherapy, radiation, hormonal therapy, the works.

A pathologist analyzes the tumor and breast tissue to identify her particular cancer cells, and the waiting time for that pathology report is excruciating. It can be three days or more to run a variety of tests on the tissue. A new test is the Oncotype DX, developed by Genomic Health, which analyzes early stage cancers that are hormone positive when there is typically no involvement of the lymph nodes. This test looks at the gene in the tumor and employs a score that helps predict the response to antiestrogen and chemotherapy treatments. This test was developed after both my sister and my wife's breast cancers, and decades after my mom's cancer. However, a friend was recently diagnosed with breast cancer, and her Oncotype DX test came in right on the line between having chemo or not. She decided to go ahead with the chemo treatment; the last thing she wanted was to be wrong on that decision.

If there are any doubts about the pathology report, consider getting a second opinion from another pathology lab. For my sister, there was never a question about her results. Initially diagnosed with a DCIS (which stands for ductal carcinoma in situ), Mary was marked as a Stage 0 patient, which meant that she had cancer cells in her breast that were confined to a duct, but had not broken through the wall. She had been having a lot of breast infections when she was breast-feeding her youngest child, Devin. Concerned that this condition somehow might be an early sign that she had breast cancer (despite all her mammograms having come back negative), she scheduled another breast exam, which finally revealed her DCIS.

The advice she received from her doctors was to get a mastectomy of one breast, since she had several DCIS sites scattered throughout like snowflakes, and no chemotherapy to follow. But she wanted a much more aggressive bilateral mastectomy, and she had one great reason: her mom had died from breast cancer, and she'd be damned if she was going to let it get her. She also had a hunch that she had inherited a mutation in either the BRCA1 or BRCA2 gene, and so she had scheduled genetic counseling and testing even before the DCIS was found. The surgeons thought she was just plain wrong. To them, she needed to have only one breast removed—end of cancer worry.

When she called me about it, I asked her what her gut said. The answer was unequivocal: bilateral mastectomy. Mary is one of those special people tapped into the universe, on almost a supernatural level, who always seems to know what is going to happen next. So I backed her 100 percent on her decision. However, her doctors didn't. Her first two breast surgeons refused to do the operation, saying it was medical overkill. So she calmly called a third surgeon and scheduled an appointment to get what she wanted. While Mary is a quiet, reflective person on the outside, she is a strong, she-warrior underneath. It's not surprising that she ultimately had her way. When Mary talks, folks listen.

Mary got her bilateral mastectomy all right, and her gut was right. It was spot-on, because in her pathology, the lab found a fully formed tumor that was missed by all three surgeons and their respective radiologists. Her sentinel node tested barely positive. "When the doctor gave me the report about my cancer, he said my cancer was on its way to the sentinel node, but never fully got there. Then he asked how I knew." And she was right about the genetic testing as well. It turned out that she was a BRCA 2 mutation carrier, and the test showed that she had a very high chance of getting cancer in her other breast, which meant that the prophylactic removal of her other healthy breast was the right call. For Mary, it was the easiest decision in the world. When I ask her if she could give me any stock tips, she just shrugs her shoulders. Bummer.

The pathologist determines if the surgeon made sure the patient has clean margins, meaning that the cancer cells are contained within the removed tissue. If, however, the cells border the edge of that tissue, then the margins are considered not clean margins or positive, and there is the risk that cancerous cells have been left behind.

The pathology report determines in what stage your loved one's breast cancer resides. Early staging—0, I, and II—is determined by the size of the tumor and whether the lymph nodes are positive with cancer or not. Stage III cancer is a more locally advanced cancer diagnosis, and stage IV, the highest stage, is when the cancer has metastasized to other parts of the body, beyond the breast and axillary lymph nodes. "Because the final pathology is not available until after the patients are discharged, and because the complication rate in breast surgery is so low; the next morning's postoperative visit is really just to review practical things like wound dressings and drain management," according to Dr. Beth Ann Ditkoff, Sharon's surgeon. "I like to see all cancer patients in the office as soon as the final pathology report is available."

Many hospitals now review the pathology report as part of a more comprehensive review of a patient's prognosis. This is often done by way of a tumor board conference, which consists of the breast surgeon, an oncologist, and a radiologist. These boards meet weekly to share information among departments, with the primary benefit that there is an integrated approach to the patient's care, and a secondary benefit that nothing falls through the cracks, medically.

Coming Home

She's coming home. Make it as easy as possible for her. There should be no fanfare, or large groups of people accompanying her. Make it as simple and seamless a transition as possible. This usually means transporting her to the hospital lobby in a wheelchair. She is going to be weak from the surgery, so wheeling her instead of walking will make things a lot easier for her, and you. Also, if she's loaded to the gills with flowers, balloons, candy, and other gifts, she can hold those items in her lap as you wheel her. Someone should always be with her when she checks out of the hospital. Ideally, there should be a second person who can get the car when she reaches the hospital entrance. If a car is not available to pick her up, then schedule a car service or hail a taxi to take her home. The hospital might provide transportation services as well.

Once she gets home, get her to head straight to bed. She needs her environment as quiet and as peaceful as possible. Make sure that she has, and takes, all the pain medications and anti-infection drugs prescribed by her surgeon. Drains and bandages will need to be changed, so offer to help with this; if you're too squeamish to do it, then ask a family member or friend to help out. Ideally, all of the incoming meals, gifts, cards, flowers, and drop-by visitors have been coordinated, as advised in the previous chapter.

Consider using a baby monitor so you can stay on top of her condition, listening from elsewhere in the house to hear if she needs anything. As she gets stronger, she'll tell you when it's time to take the monitor away.

. . . .

The Medical To-Do List

. . . .

For the first few days, everything is about medicines and drains. One great way to keep track of everything is to draft up a medical "to-do" list, which can be made on a spreadsheet or just a plain piece of paper. The list starts with her medications, highlighting what to take and when she needs to take them. Some medications might need to be injected, so if she is queasy about doing this herself—as my wife initially was—you may have to be the injector. Get a brief instruction on how to do it from the surgeon's staff; if you are uncertain when the needle is in your hand, either call someone on the staff or track down a friend who has medical experience to show you how it's done.

The medical to-do list also includes monitoring of her vital signs as well as providing when and how to change her dressings. The more organized you are with these routines and tasks, the faster she will recover. For example, the drains need to be periodically changed, with the fluid deposited in a plastic container for measurement. The amount of fluid that collects is important for the surgeon to know, as well as its color; someone needs to collect that fluid in a measuring cup and then flush it down the toilet.

There's likely to be sensitivity and pain caused by the surgery, so suggest she wear large, loose-fitting shirts. The best ones are from her husband or boyfriend. Have a wide variety of pillows in the bed so that she can elevate her body into a position that doesn't put pressure on her surgical sutures.

Given that most women are accustomed to taking care of others more than themselves, you may find that she wants to get right back into her routine—perhaps before she's recovered sufficiently. Keep in mind that it is hard for most women to just "let go" and be taken care of. They are the traditional caregivers, not you. Let her know that the roles have switched, and it is you who will be taking care of her. You are now the nurturer, and she is the nurtured. It's her needs, not yours, that matter most.

The recovery time from surgery can be up to six weeks for some major procedures. A lumpectomy has a much quicker recovery time than a mastectomy, but the actual recovery time varies from person to person. As for the emotional recovery from surgery, that has just begun and no time limit should apply.

· · · · · · · · · · · · · · ·

The Home To-Do List

· · · · · · · · · · · · · · ·

Nine times out of ten, she's already got a plan in place for you to follow on how she wants her home to operate while she's recovering. Let's face it, guys. Women are just better planners than we are. If you doubt that, just ask yourself when the last time was that you scheduled your child's camp trip, or booked your summer beach vacation house, or even arranged to have your friends over for a dinner? Exactly.

Let her take the lead on the home "to-do" list. She should still feel in charge of running her own household. With that said, there are going to be so many changes that happen after surgery that I highly recommend converting her task orders into a spreadsheet or handwritten "to-do" list, a comprehensive document that transfers all duties and responsibilities of the patient to the caregivers in her life.

The list is a hierarchical document and it covers everything and anything in her life that she has been responsible for, now passed over to you and your fellow caregivers. The list governs her life, and everyone else's life who lives in the realm of Cancer Land. It puts into grid format the daily life of your loved one, your life, and the lives of other loved ones surrounding her. It spins kids' schedules, appointments, homework assignments, and the like into one common orbit, designating where everyone needs to be each day, how they get there, how they get back. It coordinates all medical appointments with work schedules, events, even naps. It prioritizes the tasks in her life. It makes sure that everyone is fed, on time, by organizing where and how food enters the house; how lunches are made for the kids and dinners are prepared for everyone. Regarding food, consider food brought in instead of cooked in-house. She is probably on medications that make her sensitive to smell, and cooking in the house could, in fact, make her feel worse rather than better. You can also avoid this problem by closing off the kitchen, if possible. Likewise, this helps her avoid feeling guilty about not cooking for the family. She needs to be resting, not tweaking her latest recipes.

All incoming food should be coordinated, with dishes, pots, and pans identified and returned after use. This task can be assigned to the Command, Control, and Communications Officer (CCC), whose duties were detailed in Chapter 2. As part of this responsibility, have that person also set up a Family and Friends Visitation Plan that coordinates visitors and helpers. This will build a protective shield around the patient to prevent bombardment by well-wishers (and let's not overlook the curiosity-seekers). The plan creates concentric circles of access, from direct access through visits outward to Web access via support sites like caringbridge.org, which provide people with regular updates of her condition.

If she just isn't into the home to-do list concept, ask her what she needs to get done each day. If she responds "nothing," don't stop there. Suggest things that you could do for her, or get done around the house. Then, of course, you could simply do things without asking. Just make sure that when you do something, it doesn't disrupt her house. So, for example, don't rearrange her kitchen pantry or her closet. Put dishes in the dishwasher, cut the grass, straighten up the living room—knock yourself out. But whatever you do, do it the way she would want it done, not you. You can also suggest a rental movie, playing cards, or getting the kids out of the house so she can get some rest—all good stuff.

If your loved one lives alone, or doesn't have the necessary support network, she still has other avenues for help. If she is a member of a local church, for example, she can tap into its network of parishioners, who want to help members in their time of need. My sister contacted her church, and within the day she had a small army of retired ladies who cooked the meals, cleaned the house, and washed the clothes. There is also a wonderful website called Lotsa Helping Hands (http://www.lotsahelpinghands.com) that helps create an individual "circle of community" to tap local volunteers to help with logistical, medical, and personal needs. Within minutes of signing on, task and "to-do" lists can be created, and then the community members sign up for various chores and responsibilities. A "coordinator" who acts as primary caregiver spearheads the entire effort. This service is invaluable for families in which the loved one lives far away from others in the family.

········· CHAPTER 4 ·········

Chemotherapy
The Shot Felt Round the World

CHEMOTHERAPY IS THE longest part of the journey through Cancer Land, and it can be the most challenging emotionally, as well. If your loved one isn't receiving chemo, you thankfully can skip this chapter. But for many of you, this is going to be, at times, the most treacherous part of the trip. Think of the chemo treatment as a journey within a journey.

For her, chemotherapy is another major challenge to her femininity. She has already lost part or all of her breast or breasts. Now she is about to lose her hair, her appetite, her attention span, and her sex drive. If she's young, she could be facing early menopause. There is also increased risk of osteoporosis. She is going to feel tired. She might get depressed. If surgery didn't make the presence of breast cancer evident to the world, the chemo will. But chemotherapy is certainly worth all the side effects. Cancer has taken possession of her body, and so chemo's job is to evict this disgusting vagrant, for good. To do that, though, chemo must act violently against it and shut down anything and everything that it feeds upon. Chemo fights a war of attrition, killing good growth cells with the bad, like a forest fire taking out all the trees in the forest to assure that one day there will be new growth again. It's a weapon that works, and saves her life—but at what cost? As her hormones shut down, her mood swings will spike up and down faster than the stock market. She will most likely suffer bouts of forgetfulness and will be putting whatever focus she has left on herself, not you. She is going to look sick, and you are going to ask yourself what is happening to her.

You are going to feel separated from her, from life; you will be walking around in a complete daze. You are going to find it hard, and at times impossible, to concentrate. It will be harder to work, and, hell, it will even be tough to take the garbage out at night. You are going to find it more and more difficult to share your feelings with anyone, and especially her, because at certain times you will be worried you will break down like a blubbering baby and freak everyone out. So why the hell even go through with this at all?

Well, you're a man who loves your wife, mother, sister, daughter, girlfriend, cousin, friend, or coworker very much. If she weren't one of the most important people in your life, you wouldn't be reading these words right now. She is your soul mate, or your best friend, or the person who brought you into this world and who has loved you every day of your life, or she is someone who knows you better than anyone else on the planet, or someone who has been there for you whenever you needed someone to lean on. So, now it's your turn to pay her back, big time. Don't worry. You'll do just fine. Take a deep breath, hold, release—now let's get going into Chemo World.

. . . .

What Is Chemo, Anyway?

. . . .

I think of chemotherapy as some sort of *Fantastic Voyage* spaceship going through her body, a stealthy, sleek killing machine terminating all those bad cancer cells. The only thing is, there is no hot assistant like Raquel Welch inside, cruising through the bloodstream aboard the good ship *Proteus*. No, chemo is manned by a team that resembles the Orcs or the Klingons—mean, angry, strong, nasty, and damned ugly. But here's the kicker about chemo. There is as much unknown about what it is doing as there is known.

With chemotherapy, there is no way of verifying, until years later, whether it got all the cancer cells in her body. It's a very different thing from surgery. In surgery, there is an operation, a pathology report, and a course of action. When surgery is completed, there is a definitive result: how many tumors were found, how big the tumor or tumors are, whether her lymph nodes were infected by cancer cells. It's mathematical, precise, calculated.

Chemotherapy is anything but that. Sure, there is a regimen of drugs that the oncologist decides to use to fight the cancer cells. But how effective that regimen will be can't be verified until years later, unless the chemo is used before surgery, when the effects are seen immediately. Many of the oncology drugs have been around a long time, but oncologists are just beginning to learn about the new world of targeting drugs. And what they are learning is that each cancer is different for each patient. So, what works for your loved one may or may not work for the next woman. That means that new chemotherapy regimens are constantly being devised and revised with each new study published. That's why it would be impossible—no, negligent—for me to get into a detailed discussion of the various chemo treatments available; as soon as I mention one drug, it will be replaced by another. There is always a new clinical trial, a new approach, a new regimen that doctors think will work better than others.

As there is so much to process when it comes to chemo options, you should encourage your loved one to take the time to understand what the best treatment is for her, and to make sure she isn't rushed into a medical decision by her physicians. The regimen she selects is a critical decision for her future prognosis, and so it must be thought out methodically and patiently.

Likewise, picking an oncologist is like picking a partner. She is going to see that doctor for years, if not decades, so there has to be trust and confidence. My wife found out after surgery that she had ten positive nodes, three tumors, and an aggressive form of cancer at the young age of forty-one. That's rather bad news, so she wanted to make darn sure she picked the right chemo doctor. She interviewed seven of them, either in person or on the phone. She met oncologists at Memorial Sloan-Kettering, at Cornell, at Columbia, at New York University—all in New York City. Then, to make sure that the New York docs had it right, she pulled strings to get an opinion from Dr. Susan Love herself, author of *Dr. Susan Love's Breast Book,* who is a breast cancer surgeon in California. In the end, the winner was the doctor who had the best treatment regimen, which involved a clinical trial of the biologic drug Herceptin. So the doctor she picked was Dr. Ruth Oratz of New York University. Sharon explains: "I first had decided to go with Dr. Bonnie Reichman of Cornell, but Bonnie didn't have the clinical trial and Ruth did. NYU was the only hospital that had it, and Bonnie said I should go to NYU and use Ruth. So it was an arranged marriage—but we fell in love anyway."

In Sharon's case, the due diligence was exceptional. In most instances, your loved one will be fine interviewing two or three oncologists before she makes her choice. I do recommend that she meet at least two oncologists, ideally in different practice groups, so she has some comparison by which to make an informed decision.

Chemotherapy has come a long way since 1978, when my mom received her first injections. Back then, there were no effective antinausea drugs to speak of, and so my mom, and women like her, felt as if they were going to die after each round of chemo. The worst thing about this was that, with each treatment, the side effects got worse, and the cumulative effect of vomiting, vertigo, diarrhea, and stomach pains created a tsunami of anticipation torture. It was sheer hell for Mom, let me tell you.

I was never allowed to go with my mother on her trips to the oncologist, who was to me this mystical medicine man named Dr. Quan, a Chinese doctor who, in my imagination, was brewing strange potions of mold that grew on frogs from Sumatra, beetle intestines from Madagascar, and green slime from the greasy cheesesteak drippings under Pat's King of Steaks in South Philly. My sister, Mary, got to go with her, though. Maybe it was a "girl thing" back then, but neither I nor my five brothers went, except my youngest brother, Bubba, who was five at the time, who went because Mom couldn't get a babysitter to watch him. "I remember that Mom didn't want me in the back room where she got her chemo because she got so sick from it; so I was left to flip through old *Good House-keeping* and *McCall's* magazines," Bubba recalls. "She just didn't want me to see her like that. When we were driving home, she had to concentrate as hard as she could so she wouldn't get sick in the car." My dad went when he could, which wasn't often, because back in those days, employers didn't let men take off work to be with loved ones as they went through chemo unless they took vacation days. My mom told me about the Asian prints on the office walls—these fire-breathing dragons that looked right at you. She used to imagine that the dragons were the chemo coursing through her veins, burning her insides, hurting her, day in and day out. It took her three days to recover from a treatment, and she got the treatments every week, for years. Mom would hole up for days after a treatment, covered in pillows, unable to do anything, even watch TV. Then, miraculously, she would come out of her room after the third day and cook dinner.

Mom never was much of a cook, which was made worse because of the budgetary constraints imposed by the necessity of feeding seven kids. She did have the *Betty Crocker* meat and potatoes technique down pat; her meatloaf, London broil, and pot roast rivaled the best in the neighborhood. Chicken was usually baked and breaded, à la Shake 'n Bake, but we rarely, if ever, saw the likes of high-priced items like steak, seafood, or veal. I do remember that her cooking skills, limited as they were, plummeted after each chemo treatment. This couldn't have come at a worse time for our family. I was in college, two of us were in high school, two were in middle school, and two were in elementary school, all hungry, all the time. What was a breast cancer mom to do when meat prices were through the roof, thanks to OPEC's soaring oil prices? Easy. Let the meat substitute days begin with every night showcasing inventive new ways to extend a pound of meat. This was the dawning of "Hamburger Helper."

Perhaps the most legendary meat substitute meal my mom ever attempted after chemo was her infamous Baked Egg Casserole: two dozen large white eggs, cracked face up over a thick bed of spaghetti, beneath which was a thick slathering of Velveeta cheese, baked to perfection—she thought. Two major problems were not considered here. The big one was that it's never a good idea to bake Velveeta in anything at high temperatures. The second mistake was that, once attaining temperatures rivaling those of the Manhattan Project fission experiments, Velveeta transforms from its Nickelodeon orange to a volcanic blackened ash, with a grayish adhesive interior that grips everything it touches like superglue. I'll never forget my mom grabbing that living Thing out of the oven, while smoke alarms fired off in three rooms of the house. When she grabbed it with a dish towel, it was so hot that the towel caught fire, which she dowsed in the sink. Then came the really scary part: sitting down to eat it. When I looked at the dish, it resembled what I had recently seen under a microscope in my biology class—a fly's eye.

The egg yolks were a dusty white-yellow powder, the egg whites, completely black. She put a heaping pile of the "eye" on my dad's plate. The rest of us grabbed our plates and held them tightly to our chests. Neither they nor I wanted any part of it. So she turned to my dad and calmly said, "Eat it, Bill." My dad, a quiet man, a chemical engineer by trade, looked down at his fate. He took his fork, carved into the disaster, and put it in his mouth. The rest of us waited with anticipation. He swallowed, looked straight into our eyes, and said, "It's great, Anne. It really is." And then he put his fork into the "eye" for another bite. That night, William Pennell Anderson Jr., my dad, showed me what he was willing to do: anything for my mom as she suffered through her treatments—anything.

• • •

The most difficult aspect of chemotherapy for all caregivers is watching the physical and emotional struggles your loved one goes through. Sure, she has already been through a lot with her operation, but after her recovery from surgery, she is back to looking normal to most folks. But chemo is different. Chemo takes her hair away, her energy, her control over her body. It is a direct attack on her psyche and on the psyches of those around her. It is unnatural. It is a test, for her and for you, of ultimate physical, emotional, and psychological barriers. It requires a complete restructuring of her, and your, universe. Not only does she undergo a physical revolution in her body, but there is a fundamental restructuring of all relationships she has had with anyone and everyone, including you.

There is so much to take in—too much in fact, on first blush. That is why the best approach to chemo, I believe, is to view it in a free-form, open, and flexible way. Linear just doesn't work with chemo. There are too many variables and too many changes throughout the chemotherapy process that she and you have to adjust to. So, if you have operated so far in life along the straight and narrow—if you are a controlled, type A personality—it's time for an emotional engine retooling, my friend. You are in the eye of the storm; anything rigid, inflexible, and unbendable caught in the middle of that storm will break. That includes you. You are no longer an oak; you are bamboo.

. . . .

3,2,1 . . . Dripoff—Chemo Begins— The First Treatment

. . . .

I sat next to my only sister in a private chemo treatment room in Scottsdale, Arizona, as her big brown eyes swelled with tears that dripped down her cheeks. She was staring at a bag of Adriamycin, her first chemo drug, as it snaked its way through a clear tube toward her veins. The medicine's color was scarlet red. This stuff is so toxic that the administering nurse wore special gloves in order to not burn her hands if it spilled out. Adriamycin burns everything it touches outside the veins—clothes, skin, whatever. It probably would burn right through the floor that I was standing on, like that glowing green goop that came out of the monsters in the *Alien* movies that burned right through the various levels of the spaceship.

And this stuff was going to somehow save Mary's life? There had to be a better way than this.

I will never forget the expression on my brother-in-law Joe's face, as he stood in the corner, quiet as a Buddhist monk, frozen with his thoughts. What was he thinking about all this? He didn't have the experience my sister and I had had with breast cancer, and he didn't feel comfortable sharing his feelings with me. So there he stood, looking at his wife. Maybe he was praying. Maybe he was in shock. I'll never know. But he stood right beside his wife, being there for her in whatever way he could. When the red liquid began to drip into Mary's arm, she looked up at me and held out her hand. She squeezed really hard, and I held tight. She was now in Chemo Land.

I couldn't believe this was happening—again. My wife was still getting her treatments, back home in New York City. As I stared at a clock mounted on the wall, watching with too much attention to the second hand as it slid from one marker to the next, I realized that I needed to leave the room. Everyone has a place and a time where they need to be, and not be, in the caregiving process. Once her treatment had started, I had done my duty as her brother. Now she needed private time with her husband. It was Joe who was going to carry the torch from this point on for Mary, not my five brothers or dad, who had been airlifting in to be with our sis for the past few weeks. As I left the room, Joe nodded to me in appreciation.

But what happens if a loved one's husband doesn't step up to the plate for her? Well, if you're the brother, or friend, or coworker, the first thing you do is give him some time. Everyone processes bad news differently. Patience is key here, as is showing him the respect he deserves as her husband. If, however, over time, he still isn't by her side, then gentle intervention is a good idea—for her sake. If that intervention has to happen, it has to be thought out carefully. Who's the person to talk to her husband? There are many who might be the wrong person, but there's usually at least one *right* person. Perhaps that person is the patient herself; she has the most at stake here, and she always should have the final say on what happens with not only her treatment but also the support she receives. If you are going to be the one to talk to her about this, perhaps the best approach is to ask her about his involvement in a roundabout series of questions that lead her to take action and get him to be more involved. If you just tell her what to do, it may come across as patronizing, which will backfire on you. So ask things like "How is he doing when he's with you at chemo?" or "What does he say that makes you feel better?" or "What can he do to help you more?" Questions like these help her formulate the right answers that will work for her.

I'll never forget Sharon's first chemo treatment. She had always been afraid of needles—and for good reason. Nurses and doctors never pricked her veins easily when taking a blood sample. They always seemed to jab and jab before getting the needle into place. And this was just to draw a little blood. When they were finished, her arms were so bruised that they looked like she had been beaten. Now she was about to get pricked with toxic chemicals every three weeks, and she was scared about permanent damage to her veins. But fear of needles was the least of Sharon's worries. She was more concerned about whether the drug regimen would work, and even if it did, how it was going to affect her brain, her heart, and stomach. How sick was she going to be from it?

Sharon, like Mary, received the red drug Adriamycin. As with Mary, I thought of my mom when I watched the drug slide toward its target. I started crying, and so did Sharon. But Sharon wasn't thinking about herself, she told me later. She was thinking of me and what I was going through by watching yet another woman enter the gates of Chemo Hell. All she could say, over and over again as she stroked my hand, was "I'm sorry. I'm sorry. I am so sorry."

Time stands still in a chemo ward. I don't know what it is about those places. They are made to be as inviting as possible, and usually the oncology staff does a pretty good job making everyone feel comfortable. But it is a medical facility, and so maybe it's the requisite elements of being sterile and medically functional that do it. Space is often a premium in an oncology treatment office, and so your loved one will see many other women going through the same thing she is experiencing. In most centers, it's a cubicle existence, with patients separated by partitions or curtains. So the more comfortable you can make her, the better, to help her get through the time that she spends there, which is usually about an hour or so per visit.

Here are some things that you can do for her. If the center provides her with a TV and DVD player, ask what she would like to watch and then bring it along; you could play movies on your laptop for her, too. If she likes to read, offer to bring whatever book she wants. If she loves magazines, pick up a few on her favorite subjects: celebrity gossip is always a good subject in these situations, the trashier the better. The name of the game here is diversion. You want her to feel better than the ridiculous, drug-infested, DUI, bad-parent movie and rock stars. Music also helps. Sharon would listen to her favorite songs while getting her treatment, tapping her foot as the medicine dripped into her.

You can also offer to get her anything she needs. She might want water, juice, cookies, crackers, all of which are usually provided free at the center. Go get what she asks for; don't wait for the nurse to do that. When you are at the chemo center, you are your loved one's personal assistant. You wait on her hand and foot. She needs to feel that she is the queen of the chemo room. Make her proud.

Coming Home After the First Treatment

Make the trip from that first treatment to home go as smoothly as possible. If she is older, for example, don't hesitate to encourage her to use a wheelchair to make it easier to get to a car or cab. When she gets home, make sure she has everything she is going to need to assuage the side effects that the chemo will produce. For example, sometimes the drugs will cause her mouth to become dry, and she could even suffer painful sores in her mouth if she doesn't treat this dryness properly. So make sure there is plenty of crushed ice on hand for her to suck on, which helps prevent those sores from forming. She should also do regular mouthwash rinses. If she does start to get mouth sores, she can ask her oncologist to prescribe a mouthwash that helps eliminate them—it's better than over-the-counter brands. Plain warm water can also serve as a great deterrent. Her oncologist will supply her with a list of items and procedures for her to follow, which you can follow up with by making sure she is doing everything she needs to do to recover, and has everything she needs.

She should also be equipped with plenty of what I like to refer to as "distracters." After chemo, the last thing she wants to think about is cancer. Escape is an incredibly valuable coping mechanism; it helps her forget about her current medical predicament and think about something else that's lighter and more fun. For some women, distractions could be watching TV soap operas, or movies, or a romantic TV miniseries. It could be music. It could be hot baths. It could be massages. It could be knitting or meditation or Reiki. Books, if she is up for them, might work. Biographies about sick people are generally not a good idea unless they are inspirational. The best book that Sharon read during her treatment was Lance Armstrong's *It's Not About the Bike: My Journey Back to Life,* which is about his conquering of cancer and, I would argue, is about the bike, too. She also enjoyed memoirs written by other breast cancer survivors. Whatever works.

Then there is her bed, perhaps the most important home element of all. It should be covered in giant, fluffy pillows, soft blankets, and if she can afford it, high-thread-count sheets. After chemo, everything can start hurting. She might begin to suffer from intense headaches, nausea, vomiting, fatigue, dizziness. So the best place for her to go, as soon as she gets home, is bed, which becomes her Shangri-la during treatment.

What if her bed isn't such a place? Well, you need to change that—quickly. If the bed is old, buy her a new one that is more comfortable; it's one of the best things you can do for her. If she refuses, if money is tight, if she loves the bed just the way it is, then get her more fluffy pillows, a soft cuddly blanket, flowers—whatever you think will cheer her up and make her feel better in Shangri-la.

A key component to any Shangri-la is quiet. If there are young kids in the house, quiet may be difficult to achieve, but with careful planning and scheduling, it can be done. My wife and I had young kids at home—ages 7 and 5—when she went to her "La" after her first treatment. If you can get the kids out of the house at this moment (literally or figuratively), that works well. For example, if they are the right age, there is the miracle world of Disney videos to transport them. Whatever needs to be done, get it done.

You also need to make sure that she is eating right. Chemo can change her senses of taste and smell, so be flexible if tastes change. Get her foods that are going to make her happy. I suggest that, for the first week of each chemo infusion, you avoid spicy or greasy foods; she needs to know how her body reacts to the chemo.

Keeping the house clean is important throughout the chemo process. Her immunity is being compromised, so it's up to you to turn into Mr. Clean superhero. Wash with antibacterial cleaners all surfaces that she is likely to touch. Germs are her worst enemy. With that said, it doesn't mean she has to live in a bubble, but erring on the side of cleanliness will only help her.

Also, try to keep strong smells of any kind out of the house; you aren't going to know, until it is too late, what smells make her sick. Not many smells, by the way, will make her feel good, so lean toward no-smell foods. Scented flowers should be discouraged, at least during the first few treatments. Strong scents like rose or lilac could push her over the edge, and it is awfully hard to get those smells out of the house for days. The same rules apply to any and all cleaning products, perfumes, and other scents in the house—go for everything nonfragrant. The best weapon against the chemo side effects is going bland.

How your loved one reacts to chemo, in the end, is unknown until she gets the drugs well into her system and the reactions (or nonreactions) begin to take place. What is key here is how you react to her reactions. That means doing everything she wants done, as well as doing things for her that maybe she never asked for in the first place. So don't ask her if she wants you to do the laundry. Do it. Don't ask her if she wants a back rub. Start giving her one, and stop when she tells you to. Don't let the dishes sit in the sink—clean them. And never ever complain about what you do.

It's important for her, and you, to be aware that chemo compromises her immune system. She needs to be diligent in checking her temperature to make sure it is normal and alerting the doctor when it isn't. She needs to sleep and relax. This might mean keeping visitors to a minimum. If she has a lot of friends and family, everyone is going to want to be around her, to see how she is doing. Remember, though, that she doesn't need to tell them personally. You can tell them, either in person, by e-mail, or on the phone. As mentioned before, there are great Internet sites on which to post her condition. Everything at this stage in the game is about keeping the peace at home.

If you are staying at home with her during her chemo treatments, then you can help her relax. For Sharon, it was watching *The Sopranos.* Every night, we would crawl into bed and huddle together in front of my little laptop to watch what dastardly deed Tony or one of his henchmen would do to some poor unsuspecting soul who failed to pay back his debt to the family, or who challenged Tony's turf. We hadn't started watching the series until the fourth season, so she could watch as much, or as little, of each episode as she wanted, as the earlier seasons were on DVD. *The Sopranos* was the great escape for Sharon. When she got bored with that, we rented movies. I watched as many "chick flicks" with her as she desired, and in the process I got to know Bette Davis, Cate Blanchett, Audrey Hepburn, and Kate Winslet on a personal, deep level.

For my mom, my role was completely different. All she wanted to talk about was what I was up to. She wanted to know everything that was happening to me—good and bad—as I made my way through the journalism jungle of New York City. She wanted to know what it was like to meet Deke Slayton, one of the original seven astronauts in the Mercury program; at the time, I was writing an article on the commercialization of space for the *New York Times*. She also liked to gossip about the neighbors and the teachers at my brothers' and sister's schools. She loved to watch Johnny Carson on *The Tonight Show* every night, late at night, while folding laundry. When she got too tired, she'd lie down on the couch, and I would pick up the slack for her.

But the most important thing for her was to have her best friend, Caryl, there by her side. Caryl, also a breast cancer survivor, was her soul sister. They were there for each other through many a chemo treatment. It was truly amazing. So, in Mom's case, she got great solace from Caryl—more than I, my dad, my brothers, or my sister could ever give her. That's okay, too; whatever works for your loved one is her best recovery remedy.

For my sister, it was prayers to God that got her through her chemo recovery. She, like me, was raised a Roman Catholic, in St. Margaret Mary's Church in Parkersburg, West Virginia. I'll never forget how my sister, when she was four years old, thought that Jesus himself was the priest at our parish. He wasn't Jesus, but I'll be darned if he didn't look exactly like the fella up there on the cross. It was Father Patsy Iaquinta, and he wore the same big black beard and flowing curly black hair, and he even walked around town in sandals.

. . . .
Chemo: Round 2, Round 3, Round . . .
. . . .

To use a running analogy, surgery is like a sprint—hard but fast, efficient, and over quickly. Chemo is, of course, a longer run, often lasting either three or six months. Inevitably, as the treatments progress over time, you settle into a routine just like you do when running a marathon.

Chemo Land however, is such an alternative universe that it often feels like you're running to an unknown finish line. But along the way, you inevitably begin to face the big question that has been looming in the back of your mind for some time now: Why her? Well, I hate to tell you this, but the answer can be summed up in two words: don't know. There's an even better answer to this question, also in two words: doesn't matter. That's because your primary focus is on the hows and whats of making her life better, her treatments easier, her future brighter.

And when you have taken a break from doing all that, the next most important thing you need to do is turn to somebody else—someone to be there for *you*. That's right. You need a guardian angel as well—somebody you can lean on, talk to, and if you are comfortable enough, cry in front of. This advice flies in the face of all things masculine, however. Guys just don't ask for anything emotionally. That's how we were raised, how we are programmed, how we think. Well, that's total BS when it comes to this game, fellas. When you see your loved one suffering, you feel as if you are going through it yourself. And as the chemo process continues (and maybe radiation after that), you are going to find it is harder and harder to deal with. So, call your guardian angel, who usually is your best friend, and get him on your team, right here, right now.

If your loved one lives far away from your home—say, it's your sister—you are not going to have the luxury of accompanying her to most, and possibly any, of her chemo treatments. That doesn't mean that you can't be there with her in spirit. There are a number of ways you can stay in touch. For example, a phone call goes a long way to check in. If you are part of a family that is rotating in and out to be with her, then you can check in with your siblings who are on the ground with her to get the updates. If your loved one is technically savvy, she might be up for instant messaging, and even a video chat over the Internet.

If your loved one is older—say, she's your mother—there is also the concern that she get to and from her treatments safely. For older patients, this sometimes involves a bit more coordination. If she is in a retirement community, she may have access to a shuttle service. Even so, it would be good for her to have a family member or close friend accompany her to the chemo sessions. The last thing she needs is to feel more isolated and alone than perhaps she already feels.

I know that, in the case of mothers like mine, they never want their kids to know the full extent of what they are going through, probably out of some innate mother–cub programming in their brain that keeps them from putting burdens on their children. To find out what is going on, you may need to tap into alternate intelligence sources, like your dad or her husband, your sister, your brother, your siblings. It's helpful knowing the truth, so that when you are with her, you can appreciate the extent of what she is facing and feeling, and you can be of greater comfort and support than if you were acting in the dark.

Back when my mom was getting treatments, it wasn't hard to know when she was hurting because she was just plain sick. Thanks to better antinausea drugs today, that may not be the case for your loved one. If you have a good relationship with the oncologist, you might be able to get a more detailed picture of her condition, unless she throws the HIPAA laws in the way. To overcome this obstacle, just ask your loved one to put you on a list of approved contacts with whom the doctors and nurses can talk about her condition. If your loved one lives in a retirement community, there are innumerable informants ready to tell you their version of the story, including the staff and her friends there.

To really tell how she is doing, try focused observation, best achieved by listening, not talking, and watching how she moves, eats, and sleeps. You can tell what's happening if you look for the signs. When you see something is bothering her, offer to help—silently, not asking. As mentioned earlier, avoid asking what you can *do* for her, especially if it is your mom. Whenever I did that, she would say that she didn't need anything.

It's About Her Hair

No matter what she tells you, chemo is all about the hair. Don't let her fool you; women think about their hair all the time. Hillary

Rodham Clinton, speaking in 2001 to the Yale University graduating class, had this to say on the subject: "The most important thing I have to say today is that hair matters. Pay attention to your hair. Because everyone else will." If that doesn't convince you, then explain why those Hollywood stylists are paid thousands of dollars a day to arrange the tresses of Jennifer Aniston, Beyoncé, Salma Hayek, Gisele Bündchen, and Tyra Banks. Their hairstyles, after all, sell millions of magazines and generate billions for hair salons across the country.

Sometimes, a particular celebrity's hairstyle becomes The Look. Back in the 1920s and 1930s, it was all about Clara Bow and Josephine Baker, who sported the flapper bob during the halcyon Art Deco days. The 1940s, 1950s, and 1960s were all about Hollywood glamour, soft curly hair worn by sirens Marlene Dietrich, Marilyn Monroe, Rita Hayworth, Veronica Lake, Elizabeth Taylor, Brigitte Bardot, Sophia Loren, and Jean Harlow. Then Farrah Fawcett made feathered hair the rage in the 1970s, when she was chasing bad guys with a gun in one hand and pushing her hair out of her face with the other in *Charlie's Angels*. There was also Cher, with her huge hair extensions to contrast against her transparent, almost nonexistent wardrobe, while belting out "Half-Breed" and "Gypsies, Tramps and Thieves." The 1980s was the Blonde Age of Big Hair: Olivia Newton-John, Jane Fonda, and Christie Brinkley. The 1990s were all about celebrities and messy-bed-head hairdos.

Now it is your loved one's turn to sport a hair change. She has the opportunity to change a negative—the loss of her hair (which doesn't always happen, depending on her chemo drug, dosage, and treatment schedule)—into a gigantic positive. One way to do this is to hire a hairstylist at home so she can experience multiple looks as she shears her locks before her hair starts to fall out from chemo.

If she is up to the head-shaving party, however, you can help her arrange her very own "Letting Her Hair Down" event. Suggest inviting her favorite friends and family members and a photographer or videographer to document the event. Guests can bring along her favorite foods and drinks. It should be a light, fun-filled occasion during which the focus is on getting the hair cut in various styles as an upbeat, positive experience.

Be aware, however, that when it's time to cut the hair, the first snips might be upsetting to her, especially if she loves her hair just the way it is. When a woman has surgery, the scars are hidden from the public eye. But when a woman loses her hair to chemo, that effect is proof positive to the outside world that she is sick—and that she is sick with cancer. So when that first snip-snip is heard, tell her how beautiful she looks as each haircut unfolds, and remind her that her hair will grow back, and might even grow back thicker and fuller.

Some of you may want to cut your own hair, in solidarity with her. I did it twice—once for my wife and the second time for my sister. For Sharon, I cut my hair first, so she could see what I looked like bald. In other words, I paved the way for her. To take it further, I shaved my head with a razor, so that I would match how she would look when she lost all her hair. The second time that I cut my hair, I trimmed it into a Mohawk, to make the experience unique and different for my sister. (For the record, the major downside to this idea was that, when I went through airport security for the flight home, they examined everything that I owned and placed me on the Homeland Security watch list, which took me three years to get off. But it was worth every airport security delay to see the beaming grin, hugs, and kisses I got that day from my sister.)

If you feel uncomfortable about cutting your hair, that's fine, too. Do what is best for you. Some women do not want their loved ones to cut their hair under any circumstances. The last thing they want is to draw more attention to themselves by having a husband or son with a shaved head. So if she asks you to not do it, don't.

There are many women who might feel uncomfortable shaving their heads in front of their friends and family; they may want to quietly go to the haircutter alone. Then there are women who don't want to touch their hair at all. The problem with this approach is that the hair is likely going to fall out, and it generally is best for her to avoid seeing clumps of hair falling out in the shower or stuck to her hairbrush—this can be very traumatic.

If she does shave her head, whether in public or at a salon or at home, the act can be empowering for her—a symbol that she is ready to face cancer head-on (no pun intended). Let her take the lead here. Losing her hair is a reminder of her vulnerability, so respect the tremendous changes she is faced with.

How she will present herself in public after the hair is gone is totally up to her. Some women sport wigs that can be bought at specialty stores or certain hair salons. She may have a passion for scarves. She may prefer hats. Or she may wear nothing at all on her head. My sister went with a wig, not because she was uncomfortable being bald, but because she had small children and she didn't want to freak them out. My mom was a hat maniac—the louder and crazier, the better. Caryl, my Mom's best friend, also started out in hats, but then her look evolved into a traveling gypsy veil. Sharon went through all these phases, but ended up showing her gorgeous bald head everywhere she went.

Not to be outdone, I decided that I was going to own the Daddy Warbucks look and that we would assume the Dynamic Dome Duo persona. I have to admit that it created a new me. Living at the time in New York City, I acquired an air of confidence with a pinch of menace, which helped when I had to call on clients who were late paying their bills. When I dressed in my black Hugo Boss suit, with accompanying black tie, I looked like a Russian mobster, straight out of a Grand Theft Auto video game. My new aura came in especially handy when I went to Jimmy's Bronx Cafe in the South Bronx. This was a favorite haunt of mine during the chemo days, when I wanted to get away from everything having to do with cancer.

It's About Having Fun

Jimmy's Bronx Cafe was the hottest Latin club in New York City, located in the Bronx within spitting distance of Yankee Stadium. To call it a cafe was a joke. It was a club in a gigantic space that once was a car dealership. The best way to describe JB's was *Miami Vice* meets *Saturday Night Fever* meets *Salsa City*. The live music didn't start until 1 AM, so if you got there after 12:30 the line to get in would be clear around the block. Everyone dressed up when they went to Jimmy's; men wore suits, women wore dresses, period.

The first time I showed up at Jimmy's sporting my chromed head, I decided to approach the place as if my friends and I were VIPs. So, after we parked the car, I told them to walk right behind me, like a gaggle of geese, and not stop walking, no matter what happened. Very soon I was staring down two huge bouncers, sporting the widest shoulders I had ever seen in my life. They were bald, just like me. I kept walking, full speed, toward the rope. The rope lifted. We were in. Bald is a beautiful thing.

Sharon and I began to really enjoy our new clean pates. Since we both worked for our company, The Farm, we would show up for meetings in clothes that gave us a downtown, Eurotrash look, which left our clients baffled about what our "deal" was. Sharon loved to wear yellow glasses shaped like those of Edith Head, the longtime Vogue editor. (Edna Mode, the fashionista character in Pixar's *The Incredibles* is based on her.) One time, we were meeting with the marketing team of the New York Knicks; they wanted us to do a television advertising campaign for them. We walked into a conference room filled with sports jocks dressed in suits, sitting around a table cut from the center court of the old Madison Square Garden arena, with a gigantic Knicks logo in the center. We were dressed in black, head to toe, with heads white as a baby's bottom. I was beside myself, thinking that we were going to be working on this project. I had grown up a Knicks fan, had followed them on TV and in the newspapers as an impressionable kid from West Virginia. You'd think that I would have been pulling for Jerry West, a native hero from my "Almost Heaven" state, but I loved the heart and passion of Willis Reed's playing on a bum knee; I loved Clyde "The Glide" Frazier, Earl "The Pearl" Monroe, Bill Bradley, and Dave De-Busschere. I stood in marvel at Willis Reed's jersey on the way in, and I desperately wanted to touch the signed ball of the last Knicks Championship team—1973—secured in a glass case.

The Knicks marketing staff, meanwhile, took one look at Sharon and me, and their jaws dropped. After we sat down, one of the

Knicks executives discreetly leaned over in his chair to whisper in my ear, "Do you guys know anything about basketball?"

It's About Beauty Emanating from Within

In public, it was clear Sharon felt comfortable with her bald head. Not every woman is comfortable being bald, however. My sister wasn't. My mom certainly wasn't. But in the middle of Sharon's chemo treatment, we were working on a national public service campaign for Lifetime Television, "Stop Breast Cancer for Life." The goal was to encourage women to get their breasts checked, either by self-exam, by their doctor, or via a mammogram. The focus of the campaign was not only to have women get checked for cancer but also to show women that there not only is life after breast cancer but that it is beautiful—as evidenced by a group of beautiful breast cancer survivors whom we shot for the campaign.

I wanted Sharon to be in the campaign, but she was worried that, by appearing bald, she would scare some women who were already afraid to get a mammogram. So she refused to do it. She wasn't going to be in the spot—no way, no how. So I called in my heavyweight—Caryl Spease, my mom's best friend and breast cancer survivor extraordinaire.

Caryl was the first person Sharon called when she was diagnosed. Even though Caryl had met Sharon only a handful of times, Caryl dropped everything she was doing in rural Pennsylvania and came straight to New York to help Sharon get through her treatment and her first rounds of chemo. So when it was time to do the breast cancer spots, I knew where I wanted Caryl to be in them—front and center. When I told Caryl that we still needed to get Sharon in the Lifetime spots, Caryl told me not to worry.

The shoot for those Lifetime spots was a testament to the incredible willpower of breast cancer survivors. That day, the air-conditioning unit in the film studio broke down; it was a hot, muggy, high-nineties summer day in New York City. Inside the studio, the temperature climbed above 110 degrees, thanks to the giant lights we needed for the shoot. The gaffer—who is the person who handles the lights and electricity on a film shoot—warned me that at some point around 120 degrees, which we were not far from reaching, the sprinkler system would come on and that it didn't look like the air-conditioning unit was getting fixed anytime soon. I explained the situation to the women and asked if any wanted to leave. Not a single one did. So we shot and shot and shot, take after take after take. The sprinklers never turned on, but the faces of all our breast cancer survivors sure did, despite the fact that they had to be patted down by makeup artists after every take to remove all the sweat pouring down their cheeks. The end result was an Emmy-nominated campaign that is some of the best work Sharon and I have ever done together (if our kids are reading this part, don't worry, you topped it).

It's About Enjoying the Little Things in Life

Whenever she's up for it, get your loved one out of the house and take her to the places that make her feel real good about life. Her favorite restaurant is a great start. Sharon had two places that she loved for me to take her. Las Brisas is a funky Mexican restaurant in Westchester County that sports four tiny booths and six counter stools. The bathroom is in the back, through the kitchen. She loved the chicken enchiladas because they had, hands down, the greatest verde sauce and corn tortillas outside of Mexico. Our kids loved this place, too, so it was our weekly hangout. The ritual was as follows: the kids would pick out their lollipops and candy for dessert at the little bodega across the street, while I picked up the quart-sized Dominican El Presidente beer, which my wife and I would then share at the restaurant. This weekly treat put our family back into a routine we had enjoyed for so long before the cancer; now it seemed as if nothing had happened at all. Las Brisas, or "The Breezes," allowed us to drift back to the simple, uncomplicated precancer life.

As I've stated, though, there is no full return to your past. So much has changed. But not all those changes are bad ones. Sharon's favorite place of all to go was Prune restaurant, in New York City's East Village. "Prune" is the nickname of owner/chef Gabrielle Hamilton from when she was a kid. Gabrielle cooks whatever she wants, whenever she wants, and her customers are the beneficiaries. An early adopter of cooking with local produce, Gabrielle was on the forefront of transforming comfort food into gourmet fare, serving sweetbreads alongside devilled eggs, or succotash with lamb chops eaten with a spoon. Prune is truly Sharon's home away from home, what she refers to as her "happy place." It's where she loved to meet her friends, gathering strength from their support as her cancer treatment progressed. Gabrielle liked to sit Sharon either by the kitchen or at a special private area called "The G Spot," where she could keep an eye on her favorite customer. During one visit, when Gabrielle knew that Sharon was having a hard time, she had an idea: if Sharon always had to be "naked" in front of people, maybe it would make her feel better to see the chef and her staff a bit vulnerable, as well. So, unbeknownst to Sharon, me, or any of our friends, the entire Prune staff went into a small office, to emerge several minutes later without their clothes (other than their underwear). Sharon loved the gesture and broke into tears, moved by such a symbol of support.

When my mom lost her hair from chemo, she decided to have some fun with her doctors. This was back in the day when physicians often acted like gods, and patients had to obey. Well, Mom was going to have none of this baloney, as she would say to me—maybe because she had a master's in nursing, had worked for years in the ER, and had seven children who knew enough to always listen to her or else. So, after an argument with her oncologist about the chemo, she wanted to put an end to their "clowning-around nonsense." She and Caryl pulled their sewing machines out of the closet, went to the fabric store, and began sewing. The nurse called for "Anne Anderson," and two clowns stood up, sporting huge red shoes, pants, and coats; white faces; red fuzzy hair and red noses; and for my mom, a bright and shiny bald head. Her oncologist never did any more "chemo clowning around" with her again.

It's About Laughter

My mom sure had a wicked sense of humor. And she had the sharpest wit I have ever encountered. However bad she felt after a chemo session, she was never sick enough to not have a laugh about something. One day, when she was feeling extra bad (being blasted mercilessly by her oncologists because she was fighting off her second recurrence), she was in bed when I brought her a get-well card from my then girlfriend. This woman was an aspiring writer in New York City, so she wrote a poem to my mom, and accompanied it with a charcoal drawing of a tree of some sort. The drawing was well done, actually, but the charcoal made the card black and smudgy on the front, which my mom was pretty confused about—given that it was, after all, a get-well card. But she appreciated the gesture and put on her reading glasses to read the poem out loud to me. I can't recall how the actual poem began, but the theme was about the tremendous difficulties that life threw at my mom by having cancer, and how this healthy twenty-four-year-old single woman understood everything that a fifty-ish, three-time cancer survivor with a houseful of kids was going through. And then came the line: "Life is like twisted roots and gnarled stems."

This line stopped my mom dead in her tracks. She looked up at me, peering over her glasses with those razor-focused eyes of hers: "So which one am I?" she asked. "The twisted roots or the gnarled stems?" That was the beginning of the end of my relationship with this aspiring writer.

It's About the Cancer Land Leave Pass

It is important, when you are in Chemo Land, to take a break from the journey. As a caregiver, you need to find a little rest stop of your own, where you break routine and recharge your batteries. You need to find, for yourself, some form of a Cancer Land leave pass. This doesn't mean that you don't return to your post. It simply means that you step away to regain your strength so you can carry on.

You should clear your pass from Cancer Land with your loved one before you head out, because you don't want her to feel abandoned. But if she's like my wife, mom, and sister, then you won't have any problem getting "permission" to go. That's all fine, you say, but where do I go? The break doesn't have to be a big thing. You can ask your best buddy to join you for a beer, a round of golf, a run in the park—anything to get you out of the house and away from thinking about cancer, cancer, cancer. Then again, it's always better if it *is* a big thing. A client of ours, ESPN, wanted to know if there was anything that she could do for us as we went through chemo. It took me only about two seconds to think of what that might be:

"How about the World Series?" I asked.

Well, this wasn't just any old World Series I was asking about. It was the 2001 World Series, between the New York Yankees and the Arizona Diamondbacks—the same World Series that was delayed because of the 9/11 tragedy. I wanted to go to The Stadium (Yankee fans will understand and appreciate the need for capital letters here) like nobody's business. Indeed, it was where every New Yorker wanted to go to forget, for just one night, that horrific terrorist attack on the World Trade towers just seven weeks before. Twelve hours after I put in the request, I was staring at a bike messenger, who was asking me to sign for the envelope he was holding in his hand. The envelope contained two lower box seats, third base side, Yankees v. D-backs, October 31, Halloween night.

When I called Sharon to tell her the incredible news, she didn't want to go. It wasn't that she didn't like the Yankees; she loved 'em. She just couldn't deal with being in a public place so soon after not only 9/11 but also the anthrax scare that happened one week later (when four letters were sent to the New York offices of ABC News, CBS News, NBC News, and the *New York Post* containing deadly anthrax bacteria). It certainly didn't help that the game was on Halloween night either. She was worried this was a perfect place to have another terrorist attack, and she'd been through enough already, thank you very much. But I was free to go—with whomever I wanted to take. I had just been handed a golden Cancer Land Leave Pass.

I went to the game with Mac Premo, a film director and artist who worked for my company and is, hands down, the most rabid Yankees fan anywhere. His dad is a born-and-raised Bostonian, and he was *still* a pinstripes man. That takes real guts. Game 4, our game, was the one after President George W. Bush threw out the first pitch, but it still had the swooping bald eagle's landing at the pitcher's mound. It was also the second time Irish tenor Ronan Tynan sang "God Bless America" (which made the song a staple for all seventh-inning stretches at Yankee Stadium thereafter). But when you looked out into center field, you saw the tattered flag recovered from the World Trade Center. Nothing symbolized more the fragility of life. But these thoughts vanished with the first pitch. I had entered the Great Baseball Escape.

The Yankees had fallen behind 3–1, with two outs, bottom of the ninth, when Tino Martinez, the Yankees' first baseman, stepped up to the plate. Tino up to this point in the Series had gone 0–9. If the Yankees lost this game, they would fall behind 3–1 in the Series, an almost impossible deficit to overcome. There was a runner on base, so there was a chance, but the way Tino had been batting, you could feel the air going out of a lot of Yankees fans. But not me. I believed. I was sick of bad news. It was time for the fates to go my way, darn it. I had seen too much pain and suffering in chemo clinics, in the rubble of the World Trade towers downtown, in the photos of missing people posted on walls. It was time for a change, and the time was now.

When I heard the crack of the bat, I stopped breathing. When Arizona's All-Star, five-time Golden Glove center fielder Steve Finley went climbing up the wall, I prayed. He somehow pushed off the wall to elevate to a height six or more feet above it and reached for the ball. Not far enough. When he came back down to earth, he had nothing in his glove. Another miracle in the Bronx had just happened, and I was right there. Thank you, ESPN. Thank you, thank you, thank you. And as if that weren't enough, a second miracle occurred in the tenth inning, when the scoreboard, right under that tattered World Trade towers flag, lit up the night to declare, "Welcome to November baseball"—something that had never happened before in the history of major-league baseball. Derek Jeter came up to bat to face Byung-Hyun Kim, and quickly fell behind in the count 0–2. Jeter kept fighting off Kim's nasty pitches, until, with a full count, Kim tossed a slider on the outside of the plate, and Jeter reached out for it. That's right. I stopped breathing, again. Jeter had gone 1-for-15 in the Series. But that is forgotten history because with one swing he hit the ball into the right field corner. Would it stay fair? This is what Yankees announcer John Sterling screamed as it happened: "It is high . . . it is far . . . it is gone! Ballgame over! Yankees win! Theeeeeee Yankees win!"

The entire stadium erupted into a gigantic family reunion, with everyone hugging and kissing total strangers, including the members of the New York City Police Department. If ever there was a time to hug a cop, it was that night when the Yankees had done something that had only happened three times *ever* in World Series history—win a game after trailing by two runs or more in the bottom of the ninth. As Jeter rounded the bases, pumping his fist in the air, I felt that he looked right at me when he approached third base on his walk-off home run trot. Mr. November had assured me that everything, going forward, was going to be all right.

Everyone poured out of The Stadium, and headed to the bars behind the ballpark. We couldn't stop talking about what we just saw, until we met a number of surviving firefighters of 9/11 who were there making toasts to their dead comrades. We chipped in and bought them beers and shots as they cried for their lost brothers, making us cry too, as everyone hugged again during that incredibly special night, in the shadows of the House that Ruth Built.

It's About Returning to Cancer Land

As much fun as such escapes can be, the time comes when you return to Cancer Land. Your loved one has been waiting, patiently, for your return. It's time for another treatment. It's time for her to be tired again. It's time for you to cook a meal, or have a long talk with her on the phone, or pick up some items for her at the pharmacy or grocery store, or take the kids to their playdate, or give her a ride to her doctor. If you think you have it bad, take a step back and think, for just a moment, what is going on with her. She is the one doing the heavy lifting here. She is the one who is the only person in her entire circle with cancer. So, no matter how many people show up to help, to love and support her, she is the most alone person in the room. Never forget that.

Because there are times when she is going to feel alone and isolated, you have to give her room to get herself together again. If she doesn't want to talk when you do, then don't talk. If she wants to go to a movie and have you come with her, but doesn't say anything in the car on the way, don't take it personally. However, if she continues to drift deeper and deeper into herself, then it is your duty to coax her out of her shell.

When my sister would get into these moods, the best way to draw her out would be to talk about her boys. For Caryl, my mom's best friend, she liked to talk about all the funny times she had with my mom. For my mom, she liked talking about her involvement in the girl's high school cross-country team. (She served as a team mom when my sister was a member.)

I could always engage Sharon in talks about our company, since we were business partners. But when she was going through chemo, she preferred to talk about *The Sopranos* characters and the crazy antics they pulled each week. So, tap into what she wants to talk about with you, and listen—really listen—to what she has to say, then engage in the conversation in a meaningful way. If you aren't listening, she is going to know it. You have to really pay attention here.

If she's a bit withdrawn, you can also provide her with a series of mini-surprises. Write her a card. Send her flowers. Put her favorite candy under her pillow. Call her on the phone. It's all about checking in to find out how she is doing that day. Make a fuss about her—on a regular basis. As far as the big events—Christmas, wedding anniversaries, Valentine's Day, Mother's Day, her birthday— *never* miss those, especially now.

This may sound crazy but her biggest anniversary of all might well be her Day of Diagnosis. Mark it on your calendar in double-bold ink or with two alarms on your BlackBerry. If you do something special for her on this day, she will never forget it. Just acknowledging it in a note or phone call will go a long way toward letting her know you really understand what she is going through. For something a bit more special, plan a Cancer Escape Weekend, taking her to a beautiful resort or spa an hour or two from her home.

All of these efforts—no matter how small or large—are to show your love. And love is the best medicine you can give her. "Love from everyone I knew is what got me through it all," Sharon recalls. "I never knew how loved I truly was until I got sick. The extreme nature of the appreciation and love that was shown to me was the greatest gift I've ever received (other than my children)."

For example, Sharon's friends showed their love by surprising her with the "Friendship Garden." When Sharon went off to a chemo session, six of her closest friends attacked a barren piece of our front lawn with shovels, watering cans, fertilizer, soil, and a ton of plants. In less than two hours they transformed the front of our yard into a cornucopia of butterfly plants, daisies, roses, azaleas, bellflowers, hyacinths, irises, and tiger lilies, which would bloom in succession throughout the season. When we pulled up to the house, the friends were gone, so that Sharon could experience the garden on her own terms. When she got out of the car, a sea of vibrant purples, pinks, reds, and yellows flooded her vision, while butterflies flitted all around her. Sharon reached out and touched her flowers, which for the rest of her treatment, were where she went when she needed a lift.

This is exactly the time your loved one needs her friends around her. It is when she needs to feel that she is normal, just like her friends. She needs them to feel comfortable going into her room and shooting the breeze. Another thing that friends did for Sharon was to make sure she attended every dinner party they had. Every month, the dinner party rotated to a new house. They called it the Saturday Supper Social Club, and they met on the first Saturday of every month. We didn't have to host because of Sharon's treatment, but we never missed a dinner, no matter how bad Sharon was feeling. The highlight of the night was always when Sharon and her girlfriends would sing as the Saturday Supper Club Socialettes. Those special nights kept us going through our darkest times. It is those moments, with friends and family, in which to find joy in your life, in whatever form it takes.

It's About Chemo Brain

There is so much that you can do to cheer her up between chemo sessions, to rally her spirit and energy, but in the end you must remember that she is going to be tired—worn out and severely challenged. The chemo is also going to have a major impact on her moods, so give her a wide berth. The impact of the chemotherapy on her may feel, at times, as if your loved one is being rewired, right in front of you. Her hormones are out of whack. Her fast-growing cells are being killed alongside the cancer cells. Her white and red blood cell counts are being roller-coastered. And then there is chemo brain.

"It felt like I was just ditzy all the time, and slow," Sharon recalls. "Words wouldn't always come. I forgot things I was supposed to be doing or things people did or said. It was very, very frustrating. And it took a very long time to get better." This is the brain's biochemical reaction to the chemo drugs. Irritability builds, as do difficulties in memory, concentration, and clarity. She gets more and more spacey. And this happens often when least convenient, such as when her kids need her the most. When Isaac, our five-year-old, saw his mother staring out into deep space, he would get impatient, stomp his feet, and say "Mommy, stop thinking about the *cancel*!"

The deeper into chemo brain she goes, the more delicately you must navigate her emotions. Just accept her for where she is at this time—in another place. Grin and bear it, and love her. Showing her your love is the best thing you can do. And tell her she looks awesome. According to Sharon, "they loved me, they laughed with me, cried with me, indulged me, told me I looked great, that I was amazing, that I was inspiring, and I believed them. Ha. What a sucker. But it worked."

Being There as a Husband

. . . .

It's not easy being there for your wife, taking care of her; if you have kids, you are taking care of them as well. Indeed, you are now, most likely, the primary caregiver. So, when you get fed up doing the grocery shopping, the laundry, the cooking, the cleaning, the carpooling, the homework, and the bills, just remember one thing: this, too, shall pass and you will one day get your partner back. It may be six months, it may be a year, it may be longer; but in most cases, she is going to beat this disease. After enough time has passed—crazy as it sounds now—you will be closer to her than you were before this happened. So hang in there, have a beer, soda, or iced tea (whichever you prefer), and keep up all the good work. She sees what you are doing, and she appreciates it—a lot.

If you have children, then your involvement with them and their daily lives grows exponentially, since she is not going to be available as much as she was before treatment. Kids will be going through a lot in trying to process what's happening to their mom. Most of them will be fearful, and they will be good at hiding that fear. There's a belief out there that the best way to handle this situation is to not tell children about their mom's diagnosis and treatment. Nothing could be further from the truth, because kids then only imagine the worst.

Our oldest son, Seth, age 7 at the time, began to associate the takeout meals with the idea that something was wrong. He would throw a fit when meals arrived and refused to eat anything. To convince him that either Sharon or I cooked the meal, we would have friends sneak the food into the refrigerator in our own Tupperware. But when he saw it was food that he hadn't seen earlier, he would ask, "Who made this?" Lying to him would have been the worst possible response because, if he caught either my wife or me in a lie, we would lose his valuable trust in this very rocky world he lived in, raising his fears even higher.

Before Sharon's cancer, Seth loved going outside and being with his best buddies. But now that his mommy was sick, he refused to leave her side. Clearly something needed to be done. Sharon made an appointment with a counselor at the breast cancer center where she was being treated, and that counselor solved the puzzle. It turned out that Sharon was always putting on her "happy face" for Seth, that everything was not only fine, but great. He instinctively knew, however, that this wasn't the case—especially when he saw her bald head and constant fatigue. Seth was just plain worried that his mom was going to die while he was asleep; he had nightmares that, when he woke up, his mom would be gone, forever. Penny Damaskos is a counselor at Memorial Sloan-Kettering who specializes in the emotional issues faced by cancer patients and their families. Sharon explains, "Penny told me what I had to do, and it was the hardest thing that I've ever done in my life. I had to promise Seth that if I was going to die, I would tell him by giving him plenty of advance notice. The very next day, he left my side and went out the door to play with his friends. It was amazing."

Kids need to know that everything is going to be fine; and if not, they need to know the bad news at a level appropriate to their age. But the most important thing that you can give them during this difficult time is routine. Keeping things normal around the house sends the message that, no matter what else is happening, or will happen, they are going to be cared for, everything is going to be fine, and life is going on just as it always has.

Some kids never seem to have any problems whatsoever. Our youngest son, Isaac, age 5 at the time, didn't have a problem with the fact that his mom had cancer; in fact, he was pretty darn proud of it. One day he got into an argument with another five-year-old girl during a playdate. She started to argue with him that her dad had a cold, and so he was much sicker than Isaac's mom because he was sneezing and blowing his nose all the time. That day, Sharon was wearing a bandana, wasn't coughing or with any other apparent symptoms, so the little girl thought Isaac was being ridiculous. Isaac's response? "Yeah, well my Mom's got cancel," and then proceeded to yank Sharon's bandana off her head, exposing her bald pate, to the horror of the little girl. Her eyes grew to the size of saucers as she stared in shock. "Whaaat Haaaaaapppeenned????!!!!!"

....

Being There as a Son
....

As America ages, the need for caregiving rises. Many elderly patients above the age of seventy-five rely on family members to help meet their needs at home, and in the face of this tough economy, with declining retirement portfolios, that need is only going to grow. If you live near your mom, it's important that you check in on her regularly. She needs to be cared for, and she needs her son's love.

Your mother brought you into this world, so the least you can do is bring her something that cheers her up now and then: split pea soup, handwritten cards from her grandkids, trashy magazines (never underestimate those!), her favorite movie on DVD, whatever. The key is to just spend time with her. If she lives alone, she may just need company—and a good, strong hug. She also might need her lawn cut or her prescriptions filled.

Caregiving is tireless, repetitive, thankless work. To be a caregiver worth your salt, you must be patient yet persistent in your care. You must be generous, not only with your time but also with your emotions. You must be a good listener. You must be there for her, in all ways. The reward is that you know you are helping and making a difference.

What if you live far away from her and can't come to the door when she needs you? You can visit, of course, and call frequently, but doing more than that may be difficult for you. The best alternative in this situation is to make sure that she is being cared for by others whom you trust. That could include your dad or other family members, like your sisters or brothers, aunts, uncles, or her friends. If she needs more care, you can make sure that there is good professional help available. You can regularly follow up with the agency, after talking with her to determine her needs, and establish that she is getting the best care possible that she, or you, can afford. If she does have good home care, it is important for you to show those caregivers your respect, so that this respect is passed along to your mom. But, in the end, there is no one better than you, as her son, to see her as much as you can. You are, and will always be, her baby. So be there for her, as much as possible.

. . . .

Being There as a Dad

. . . .

The best way to be there for daughters with cancer is to not only say that you are there, but to show up. This means that you go to her house, help her and her family with errands or other chores that need to be done. You make yourself available and useful. If you don't live in the same town as your daughter, this will mean making trips to see her. Her disease is a serious one, so don't treat it lightly, whatever her prognosis. And it is important for you to not only respect her treatment decisions but also support them. If she is married, never step in the middle between her and her husband.

Is it all right to show your emotions to your daughter? Sharon says of her dad, "He made me see him as the more vulnerable one. He had always seemed so invincible to me, and he was completely decimated—to the point that I could hardly recognize him. But the thing he did best was [that] he trusted me. He never questioned me or lectured me. That was really important, especially because it was him. The lack of his trying to control me actually made me feel empowered."

Being There as a Brother

. . . .

When I was with my sister, the best thing I could do for her was make her laugh. We had a lot of really good laughs throughout the chemo process, but the best one was a belly-shaker. I went with her to the waiting room at the Mayo Clinic Cancer Center. The room was huge. It felt as if we were walking into the lobby of a movie theater. There were stations of chairs, kind of modules, with the usual outdated magazines at each end of a grouping of chairs. When Mary and I walked in, I was sporting a huge rooster-tail Mohawk, spiked straight up in the air. Mary, meanwhile, had shaved her head, so the two of us looked like we had gotten lost off the set of *Mad Max*. Folks in Arizona are pretty conservative, so they didn't know what to make of us, dressed head to toe in black. To push my look over the top, I was wearing a big pair of black Doc Martens boots and my keys hung off my belt loop, which caused them to jingle as we approached the reception desk to register Mary.

As we walked through groups of people, it was if we were parting the Red Sea. Everyone just scattered. Sid Vicious of the Sex Pistols had nothing on me that day. After Mary signed in, we sat down next to a group of folks and started talking, oblivious to our surroundings. A minute later, Mary noticed something and tapped me on my shoulder. I turned and saw that no one was sitting within 30 feet of us. We looked at each other and started laughing so hard my ribs were jangling my keys even louder than before. That was a great way to start Mary's first chemo session.

Sharon's brother, David, took a different approach to humor, but it was just as effective. Even though David is five years younger than Sharon, he grew up playing with her because she needed him to move her Ken dolls around the Barbie house compound. So the two of them got into a habit of mimicking voices for various characters who would come to visit Barbie when she was either at her beach house in Malibu or at her estate in Beverly Hills. So whenever David was with Sharon during treatment, he would go right into his Ken, Barbie, and friends voice imitations, which always got Sharon laughing.

Because David lived eight hours away, he was frustrated that he couldn't be there more often for Sharon as she made her way through her chemo infusions. So he worked out a deal with her. When she was getting chemo, she had to listen to tape recordings of his voice, which he had made on a portable digital recorder that he mailed to her. As the chemo was dripping into her arm, saliva was dripping from Sharon's mouth, her long and hysterical laughs unending, as she heard his comic renditions of Tom Petty's greatest hits, sung without consonants. For instance, here's David's rendition of a verse from Tom Petty's "Refugee":

Uh-O A-ah OO-i I uh Eh-OO-EEEE [translated: don't have to live like a refugee]

Or, his version of Petty's magnum opus, "Don't Do Me Like That":

Oh oo ee I ah

Oh oo ee I ah

Uh ih I uh oo ay eee, oh oo ee I ah [translated: don't do me like that]

If tiny recorders aren't your fancy, there are many new technologies available that enable you to be "right there with her," in real time, even though you are living thousands of miles away—for instance, instant messaging, iChat, texting, Facebook, MySpace, and Twitter, to name just a few.

·················
Being There as a Friend or Coworker
·················

For a friend, perhaps the best thing that you can do for her is to be available when she needs you. She might need you to pick up a prescription at the drugstore or get her something to eat from her favorite Chinese restaurant or cut her grass—or just to talk to or watch a movie with. A friend is different from a family member: she didn't pick her family members, but she did pick you. Think, then, about what it is that brings the two of you together as friends, and then consider in what ways you can make her chemo process go that much easier, based on what you know about her as her friend.

She might say that she is doing fine, and that she doesn't need anything from you—but you will know when that isn't the case. If she says she doesn't need anything at all, suggest some things you can do for her; and if that doesn't work, then go ahead and do something without asking. If you act without her input, that's fine so long as you know that what you are doing will not upset her later.

As a coworker, what you do for her during this time is a bit trickier, because of your professional relationship. With that said, you can offer to take some of her workload if she is amenable to that and it doesn't get her in trouble with her superiors. If you are her boss, by far the best thing that you can do is cut her plenty of slack in terms of her work assignments. That doesn't mean that you have to treat her differently from her other coworkers, but it does help to be a little more flexible regarding her hours, especially if she is feeling sick from her chemo treatments.

There are, of course, bosses who just don't "get it" when it comes to breast cancer. If you have authority over a boss who is such a person, set them straight by convincing that individual that a cancer patient is still a normal, functioning person who can do her work, but who might just need a little extra room to function, especially if she's not feeling well.

I was recently told about a boss who got angry when he discovered a freelance writer on his staff lying down on a couch because she was having a bad reaction to her recent surgery—a mastectomy—an hour or so before she had a meeting with a client. The boss was worried, not about how she was doing but rather about how his client would react to "her just laying around, cluttering up the office," the boss said. He added, "She had violated a 'separation of church and state' when it comes to business and personal things, and work was no place for her to be if she was going to lay on the couch." Thankfully, this boss had a partner who stepped in and took control of the situation. The partner expressed empathy for the woman, who then attended the meeting and the client was none the wiser.

. . . .

The Last One Standing

. . . .

Know that your loved one is fighting the battle of her life. The "Thrilla in Manila" and the "Rumble in the Jungle" Muhammad Ali fights have nothing on her battle against breast cancer. It is her job to be the last one standing. It is your job, as her ring corner man, to make sure she has everything she needs to kick cancer's butt, by "floating like a butterfly" and "stinging like a bee."

This fight is a whole lot longer than a twelve rounder. It doesn't end when one combatant falls to the canvas for a ten count. It is a battle to the death. And you can help make sure she is the winner. The greatest fighter-philosopher of all time, Rocky Balboa, had this to say about what the fight for life is all about:

> The world ain't all sunshine and rainbows. It is a very mean and nasty place, and I don't care how tough you are, it will beat you to your knees and keep you there permanently if you let it. You, me, or nobody is gonna hit as hard as life. But it ain't about how hard you hit; it's

about how hard you can get hit, and keep moving forward. How much you can take, and keep moving forward. That's how winning is done.

Breast cancer is about how hard she can get hit and keep moving forward. How much she can take and keep moving forward. Most of the time, she will be crushing her opponent. But there might be a lot of hits she has to take in order to win. For example, she might have her veins collapse from all the pricks to inject the drugs that have to be put in her body. She might need surgery by a vascular surgeon to put a port (a small flexible diaphragm into which needles can be inserted) in her vein to make injecting the toxic chemicals easier. Her temperature might rise so high from an infection that she will need IV medication to bring down the fever. She might be vomiting for days, or even weeks at a time. She might have trouble breathing, and have to draw air from an oxygen tank to get her through the next round of chemo. She might need booster shots to raise her red and white blood cell counts high enough to get the next chemo dosage. She might not be able to sleep for days because of headaches, dizziness, and vertigo. She might not be able to swallow her food because of a throat irritation or lack of appetite. She might lose her sense of taste and smell.

Then, again, she might not have any of these problems, which is lucky for her, and you. But in the end, there is only one golden rule that you must follow, no matter what happens and no matter what the cost: that you will always Stand by Her.

······················· CHAPTER 5 ·······················

Warning

The Radioactive Emotional Fallout

BEFORE MY WIFE was diagnosed with breast cancer, and way before we were married, Sharon surprised me by buying a trip for two to the Cayman Islands, where we went scuba diving for a week. This was a big deal to me because I love to dive. I had been to Australia, Thailand, Indonesia, and the Bahamas. So when Sharon booked this trip, she skipped the tourist traps of Grand Cayman and secured a cute little bungalow by the sea on Cayman Brac, so that we could dive every day along the incredible cliff walls of Little Cayman. To make the trip even more special, Sharon decided to get her scuba certificate so that we could dive together.

The only thing that scared Sharon about this trip was the idea of going on a deep dive, which for recreational divers is anywhere from 100 to 130 feet down. When it was time for her to go with me, she said "No way." I convinced her to do it by telling her that, when she got below 100 feet, she would see a deep blue like she'd never seen before. Down there, in the Big Blue, color changes from a light, clear Columbia blue to a pure black. The deeper you go, the darker it gets. What is really strange in this world is that you can easily lose orientation—of what is up and what is down. There is no beginning and there is no end—just the vast emptiness of an endless ocean.

After much trepidation, Sharon descended with me into the great beyond, while holding my hand. She was fine—happy, in fact—until we got to the part of the dive where we had to enter a dark cave. On the boat, the divemaster had told us about this cave, instructing us that it might seem a bit scary, but it wasn't. The bad news for Sharon was that she could see only the entrance, not the exit, and everything in-between was dark. There was no way she was going into that cave. She was terrified, and she started to pull away from me, seemingly in a panic, as she began ascending toward the surface.

In diving, panic is without doubt the worst thing that can happen to you underwater. Scuba diving is all about remaining calm when problems arise, whether they be low air, excessive currents, lost masks or fins, or a leaky mask. You can deal with just about every situation until you panic; and the worst thing you can do, after you panic, is to shoot up toward the surface from a great depth. If you do that, you run the great risk of getting the bends. The bends, more scientifically referred to as decompression sickness, occurs when nitrogen bubbles form inside your bloodstream. The bubbles form because of the sudden pressure change caused by a rapid ascent. These bubbles then begin to circulate as tiny bombs throughout the body, rupturing veins, arteries, lungs, and anything else that stands in their way. It's a horrible way to die. The pain is excruciating, and the prognosis for survival in the case of severe bends is grim.

So when I perceived that Sharon was shooting up to the surface, I grabbed her leg and refused to let go. Given that she was a new diver, she wasn't able to control her buoyancy well, so she thrashed even harder to get away from me, because she thought that I was forcing her into that awful cave. The dive master had to wedge himself between us to stop our fight. Words spoken underwater mean nothing; if you speak underwater, all you hear is mumbling. The only way to communicate is either to write on a waterproofed tablet or use hand signals. But Sharon's signal to me—flight to the surface—scared me. I refused to let go of her, even though she stared directly into my eyes, signaling over and over in the international language, "I'm okay, I'm okay, I'm okay!!!!" But I wouldn't let go— until the divemaster made me. I wasn't going to lose her, to anything or anyone else. I learned later that her ascent hadn't been panic but carelessness. She had no idea that she was floating upward. But I had, and I had panicked that I would lose her forever, in that infinite, deep sea of blue.

. . . .

Your Deep Blue Sea of Sadness

. . . .

Your time is coming—or you may have already come to your own version of the deep blue sea. It may have happened right after she was diagnosed, or maybe after her surgery, or perhaps during her chemo. But for most men, the real deep blue moment happens some time in the later stages of chemo or when her radiation treatments begin. The deep blue sea is where your deepest fears, emotions, and feelings are trying to swallow you, to drag you into a vast emptiness of sadness, silence, and isolation.

You are alone, abandoned, lost. It's everywhere—in everything you do, touch, feel, smell, and think. It wants to destroy you, your loved one, your family, and your friends. It wants your job, your future, everything you have ever held dear. You are inside that deep blue sea, and you have no idea how you will get out. You've been swallowed, whole, by a perfect storm of unhappiness, mental pain, and deep emotional suffering. You, my friend, have been dumped overboard without a life preserver, without a paddle, and with heavy psychological weights tied tight around your ankles. You are in the Deep Blue Sea of Sadness.

Every man's sea of sadness is different. Some sail through it fine, without incident, while others, like me, struggle with its undercurrents for years. The good news is that the Sea of Sadness can be navigated; the vast majority of us make it safely through the storm. But the bad news is that calming this storm is far from easy, and takes an awful lot of openness, communication, and honesty to see your way through it. The journey is treacherous and the setbacks can be many. You will be tossed from your mental lifeboat not once but several times, as you make your way back to calmer emotional shores.

Don't expect to hear about the Sea of Sadness from a fellow male caregiver going through what you are going through. That's because he, like you, probably doesn't want to talk about it to anyone—not your loved one, not your family, not your friends, and not your co-workers. Why not? Well, it's too damn scary to expose your sadness to anyone. So you hold it inside, deep and hard, hoping that it will some day go away.

I hate to tell you this: the more you hold on to it, the more it festers, burrowing deeper into your psyche. Every day that you don't reach out to someone about it is one more day it eats away at your emotional bedrock. It's a psychological cancer, and your life, like hers, has just gotten extremely toxic. Deep down in your Sea of Sadness is a place you've never seen before. Atlantis? You wish. No, this is a place where you hope to never return to again, a place where emotional fallout spreads its poison into everything.

. . . .

Radioactive Emotional Fallout

. . . .

Radiation has got to be one of the most ominous words in the English language. It reeks—or maybe better, leaks—of decay, destruction, and desolation. Once it appears, it never seems to go away. Radiation doesn't even have a life. It has half-lives that go on and on and on, forever.

When you hear *radiation,* you may think about Hiroshima and Nagasaki. Approximately 120,000 people were killed from the nuclear bomb the United States dropped on Hiroshima, and 80,000 more died in Nagasaki from a second bomb. Most people died from the initial explosions, which sent mushroom clouds over eleven miles into the air. But many more died later on from radioactive fallout, suffering painful deaths from burns, leukemia, and other related diseases. Approximately 9 percent of all cancer and leukemia deaths from 1950 through 1990 among atomic bomb survivors were directly attributable to the radiation released by those bombs.

Say nothing and do everything. That has been the *modus operandi* for most guys in their caregiving roles up to this point. All the "bad" boiling inside you—well, you'll keep it to yourself, right? That's what a man is supposed to do, or what many of us were trained to do since we were little boys. Boys don't cry. Boys don't complain. Boys must be, well, boys.

Don't ever underestimate the radioactive fallout of emotional pain. It can, and will, get to every guy eventually, at some point during his caregiving experience. Cancer, cancer, cancer, you say—enough! You're so tired of hearing "How's she doing? How's she doing? How's she doing?"

You long to hear the question, "How are *you* doing?" And you have the answer: not well, thank you very much. Not well at all. Cancer has taken over everything in your life, and not in a good way. Your relationship with her, with your job, with everything in your life has become more intense, more stressful, and therefore harder to deal with on a daily basis. So whatever isn't going well with you just gets worse—all thanks to *c-a-n-c-e-r*, the prime-time sponsor of misery and pain. Cancer is to you what Kryptonite is to Superman: it brings you to your knees. It's what makes you *so* angry; in the way gamma rays caused an enraged Bruce Banner to transform into the uber-muscled Hulk. Cancer has turned you against your own self, maybe in a way that a radioactive spider bite turned Peter Parker into Spider-Man. Wait a minute. Superheroes. Radiation. Cancer. What does this have to do with my life?

Everything.

You are her superhero. And so you must begin your next, and perhaps most important quest of all: to do battle, one-on-one, with your arch nemesis—yep—your radioactive emotional fallout.

Emotional and Sexual Fallout as Her Husband

She's tired. She's emotional. She's distracted. She's nauseous. She can't think about it right now. She's not interested. She's just not into it. And all you can think about is one thing, and one thing only: when are we ever going to have sex again? If this hasn't been a problem up to now, then you're lucky. That doesn't mean that it isn't coming. It usually happens to most husbands at this stage in the cancer treatment process. The thing is that it's not always her fault; it might be yours.

Let's first explore if it's your problem. How many of you have hesitated to touch her because you are worried about how she will react? Maybe she is embarrassed by her body, and she doesn't want you to see her the way she is now. Maybe you are worried that you are going to hurt her in some way by touching her. Maybe you are worried about how you are going to react to her scars. You don't want to hurt her feelings, so you stay as far away from her as possible when it comes to intimacy. If she tries to become intimate with you, you have many reasons to give for why it's just not the right time. You're tired. You're distracted because of things happening at work. You heard your kids in the other room. You need to make a phone call to your brother on the West Coast.

And what if it's her problem? She doesn't want you to see her changed body. Her sexual drive is very low. She is in pain, often. She might be going through early menopause, thanks to chemo or hormonal therapy, so the last thing that she wants is to have sex with you when the result is pain caused by chafing and vaginal dryness. She is often or always tired. She wants to talk with her friends, family, or coworkers on the phone or in person, right now. She wants to reconnect with her kids when she has a bit of energy. That leaves little or no time for you. How do you react to all this?

Many of us turn to the stiff-upper-lip technique. When she asks how you are doing (and all you can think is the mantra "sex, sex, sex, sex") you say two- and three-word sentences like "I'm okay," "I'm fine," "All's well," "No problems here." Meanwhile, inside, a bubbling cauldron of testosterone is building, building, building—

getting hotter, meaner, nastier. Think of the Orcs as they work in the mines of volcanic lava, preparing weapons of endless destruction. Then you start hearing the angry, resentful questions percolating inside your brain, which you have no answers for: "Why doesn't she ever pay any attention to me?" "Why doesn't she want to have sex with me?" "Isn't she attracted to me anymore?" "Does she even care?"

Jill Taylor-Brown, director of Patient and Family Support Services, CancerCare, Manitoba, Canada, calls this "the moment when husbands and wives going through breast cancer treatment have a sexual standoff. The woman wants the man to initiate intimacy to [make her] feel she is desirable. He is waiting for his wife to show intimacy signals because he doesn't want to come across as pushy." This leads to emotional separation. Her intimacy is often emotional—touching, coddling, cuddling, spooning. His is physical—sex, sex, and more sex. The two sides, battling for position, cross each other out, leaving each other rejected, angry, and withdrawn.

So, for us guys, we try to further internalize this struggle, telling no one in order not to worry or upset her. But whenever we try to say one thing to our wives so that there is no trouble caused, but inside think and do something else, then bad things are probably going to happen. Turning bad is not a good thing for her or you at this stage in the treatment process, but the temptation is going to be there—greater, perhaps, then ever before in your lifetime. That's because the easiest thing for you to do right now is to escape from all the cancer crap you have been dealt. You want to hit the road, run away, and embrace any and all bad-boy tendencies you once had, never had, still have, or want to have. Guys are, after all, biologically wired to roam, to explore, to experiment, to discover. If it's bad roaming, exploration, experimentation, and discovery, this could turn into activities like drinking, gambling, Internet porn, sex with another woman, or drug abuse.

Susie from Texas, in the middle of her cancer treatment, often found her husband passed out, completely incoherent, on the floor, naked, after he refused to come to bed with her. This happened several times a week. But that was just the beginning of his bad-boy behavior. When he wasn't wasted, he turned to online gambling—in a big way—losing tens of thousands of dollars of their money, which had been earmarked for important things like college, family vacations, and food for the week. "I would have been less mad at him if he were screwing around on me, [rather] than being so stupid with our money," Susie said. "I had taken time off from my job to be treated, so money was tight. And this bastard was just pissing away our money." Susie is still married to her husband, but she remains furious with what he did, not only to her but also to her children's future, by gambling it away. Their future as a family is not sound.

I know that you are telling yourself that you could never do anything like this, especially given her vulnerable situation right now. But you should never underestimate your bad-boy feelings. They are right there in times of stress, desperate to act up and act out. This often happens when she is as far away from you in terms of sexual desire and intimacy as possible. With breast cancer treatment, her sexual prowess has been kicked to the curb. For one, her estrogen and testosterone hormones are behaving like bad stocks in a bearish stock market. With menopause, not only has her desire dried up, but her vaginal fluids have as well. So for her to have sex with you, it could be painful; but there is a solution—lubrications such as Astroglide, Sliquid, Liquid Silk, or K-Y Liquid. Mentally, with treatment-induced menopause, she is forced to face the fact that she is growing older at the same time as she is facing a life-threatening disease. This is a tough combo to handle. You, meanwhile, are probably showing no sympathy because all you want to do is get some sexual satisfaction. Not good for her; not good for you. Result—a standoff.

This is complicated by the deep emotional struggles she's facing to accept her new body. Her femininity, in her mind, has been compromised, challenged, and for some women, totally crushed. If she has had a lumpectomy, her breast has been scarred; if she has had a mastectomy, she has lost her breast or breasts. She now is missing a major physical part of herself that defined who she has been as a woman. An integral, invaluable part of her has been taken. Gone. Forever. If you, in any way, think this isn't a big deal, think just for a moment how you would feel if you no longer had a penis. How important is it for you to be a man? Why would it be any different for her?

With her loss of breast or breasts usually comes a loss of sensations—loss of the physical sensation of a breast being there, and lost sexual sensation from stimulation of her nipple. Now, all she feels there is numbness or pain. So, this is what she is feeling when she looks into your blank stare, as you tell her everything is okay, fine, no big deal, thumbs-up.

• • •

Intimacy is not the only emotional fallout concern. There is, for example, the problem of total burnout that comes with extensive caregiving. You hit a wall, and the last thing that you want to hear, or talk about, is her. Yet, over and over again, all you hear is "How's she doing? How's she doing? How's she doing?" while no one is asking, "How are you doing?"

If you are suffering from burnout, everything and anything, no matter how small, seems to get in your way. It might be when you come home after a hard day at work and see the dishes piled up in the kitchen. Or maybe the kids aren't doing their homework because she wasn't pushing them. It could be the bills, piling higher and higher, not paid or even touched until you sort through them. Maybe it's the refrigerator, which hasn't been cleaned lately, or the dog hasn't had a bath and smells like moldy towels. The garbage can is overflowing. Your teenage son didn't cut the lawn. Your daughter's dollhouse and all of its innards are scattered up the staircase, down the hall, into her bedroom, and all over her closet. Dinner isn't ready, not even started.

You see all of this while your wife is sitting there, telephone to her ear, having a meaningful and important conversation with her friend—for maybe the last hour or much longer. You want to break something, anything. Meanwhile, you are breaking down inside—sometimes completely, as I did.

Sharon remembers that time: "The hard stuff between us kicked in during chemo. My weakened state meant that John had to do so much more of the work around the house (already a problem between us), and I felt guilty about that. He would often be surly and angry about it, but when I would ask him to talk to me about it, he refused. Meanwhile, his mood was very dark. I called his friends and begged them to take him out so he could vent with them (since he wouldn't with me). John seemed to hate the fact that he had such a thankless job (as a caregiver). I was constantly thanking him for all that he was doing. But then I would get up the next day and people would ask him how I was doing all day long, and not him. That just made him even angrier. This all culminated on our 'getaway' trip to Montreal to try and fix things between us."

Canada, however, didn't fix anything—it just made things worse. You'd think that going for a long weekend to a city steeped in French culture, festooned with all the love trimmings—romantic restaurants, wonderful little boutique shops, French food and wine—would be just the ticket to get me out of my funk. But every time I saw a cute couple kissing each other on a street corner, holding hands as they walked down a cobblestone street, or laughing uncontrollably at each other's bad jokes over a steaming bowl of caffe latte, I kept wondering why Sharon and I had been robbed by cancer to live a life of fear, anxiety, and pain.

When Sharon would complain about being tired, or an ache or pain (understandable given all of her chemo drugs and radiation treatments), I would:

1. Roll my eyes

2. Let out a good huff or two of frustration

3. Demand that she pick up her walking pace as we toured the city

4. Storm away from her in anger

In trying to remember what I went through during Sharon's breast cancer treatment, I found that some events were much harder to recall than others. The "Montreal getaway," though, came rushing back to me in sharp and painful detail. I clearly remember being on one of those half-bus, half-boat contraptions called the Amphibus, which by the way was the first of its kind in the world. I was sitting next to my wife as she reached for my arm to lean on my shoulder, while we gazed at this bizarre stack of concrete apartments, a world-famous structure called Habitat '67, built as a city of the future for Montreal's 1967 Expo.

To me, in my angry state of mind, it looked like a jumbled mess, just like my life. When we got off the boat, Sharon wasn't feeling well, suffering from a bit of seasickness. She was woozy from all of the drugs, coupled with the fact that she hadn't eaten in awhile. As we walked down the street, she stumbled, then fell. So what did I do? I left her, right there in the street. I couldn't take it any longer. I had flatlined. I left her and I didn't look back. I just started walking, to get as far away from her as possible. When she got up, I was gone, and she stood on the corner, crying and furious with me because I had essentially abandoned her.

I was feeling sorry for myself, and I didn't want to be with anyone, especially her. I started wandering aimlessly through the streets of Montreal. There was some festival in town celebrating Canada's Native American culture. I found myself surrounded by celebrants, dressed as Indians, handing out cornhusks, beer, and trinkets to the oncoming tourists. I knew better. Native Americans weren't happy back then, and they certainly weren't happy toward white men who had looked just like me. I wanted to get away from all people and everything and anything that had to do with humanity. When I found a big patch of dried cornstalks off in a corner, I sat on top of it, and looked up at the gray sky. I realized that I was lost, in Montreal, with no way home.

Sharon, meanwhile, limped to the closest building, a hotel, where she sat in the lobby for a very long time. "Something really died in me that day—I have forgiven it, but will never, ever forget it," she said. "It confirmed to me that John had very real limits as to how understanding he could be. Even though I couldn't control being sick (or being so light-headed that I fell down), his anger took him away from me when I needed him, and I had to face that reality alone on top of facing my illness. I can see why some couples don't make it through an illness like this."

Emotional Fallout as Her Son

When I think about all the emotional fallout moments with my mom while she was going through breast cancer, I'm reminded of a joke about the difference between Catholic guilt and Jewish guilt. Catholic guilt is for all the things that you shouldn't have done, but did, and Jewish guilt is for all the things that you should have done, but didn't. My mom, a born and raised Roman Catholic, was some-how able to implant both guilts deep in my psyche (maybe that's why I, a baptized Catholic, married a nice Jewish girl). I had failed both for what I hadn't done and what I had done, which resulted in a staggering one-two stab by my dear mom, straight to the heart. Here's what was really happening:

Anne Anderson was playing her martyr role to pure perfection. She never wanted anyone to help her, but then she had no problem complaining, as she went about the house doing chores, that no one helps her. Whenever I came home to help her around the house, she got mad at me for not coming home sooner. And then when I started to help her—cleaning, washing the clothes, shopping for groceries, whatever—she would make me feel that I couldn't do anything the right way, which made it twice as hard for her because she would have to do it all herself. It always began with a "woe is me, no one helps me, I can't take this anymore scenario," but as soon as you tried to do one thing for her—just one—she would pull out her Joan of Arc sword and attack you for being so insensitive to the fact that she is not a cripple, that she can handle everything, and thanks but no thanks for your help.

I had entered a new field of battle. Only this time the battle wasn't with the cancer, but instead with my mom. She was fully armed and ready to kill me with her Cancer Weapon. Here's how the Cancer Weapon works. Whenever you get into any type of disagreement with your mom, you lose. It could be about how you are helping her—or not. It could be about her doctors, her treatment, how she's feeling. Whatever you say, it's wrong. And when you refute that, she hits you over the head with one simple fact: you don't have any idea what you are talking about, and she does because she has cancer, you don't, and you will never understand. She has just plunged that weapon straight through your solar plexus.

Moms use the Cancer Weapon as a way to regain control over their lives. So when my mom attacked me for not properly separating the whites from the colored clothes or folding them the exact way she wanted them folded, she did it the way she talked to me when I was her little boy. She, meanwhile, was Mom with a capital M.

What do you do when your mother is wielding this weapon everywhere? You tell her that there is no way you can help her now, and you walk away, calmly and nicely, promising her that when she is ready to accept your help, she should give you a call. This approach is respectful to her and neutralizes the manipulations immediately. When I tried this with my mom, she burst into tears and then asked me to help her fold the towels—a perfect compromise.

When your mom is going through breast cancer, there comes a time when you think that, maybe, this is how she is going to die. It then makes you think about your own mortality. Our moms, throughout our developing years, were the bedrock of our existences. The sun came up when our moms said it did. Life without mom? Unimaginable. Yet breast cancer has forced us to think about it. And this is happening while the outside world doesn't fret over your conflicts with your mom. Plus, you probably also have many other pressures—at work, at home with your wife, girlfriend, significant other, kids, and so on. If you are living at home with your mom and dad, and you're reading this, you are probably a college or high school student who is trying to get good grades, to get a good job, or to get into a good college, and the last thing you need right now is for your mom to go through all this. It's just not fair to you, or her. And it isn't fair. But it is what you, and she, have to deal with.

If your mom is older, say in her seventies, eighties, or nineties, you and your other siblings might be involved in her financial situation. How has she paid for her treatment up to now? How will she pay for it in the future? Does she qualify for Medicare, Medicaid, or some other federal, state, or local program that could help her out? Speaking of other siblings, how are they weighing in on her situation? We were all raised to think that brothers and sisters should pitch in for everything equally, a share-and-share-alike mentality. But, in most cases, mentality and reality operate separately. The reality is that some siblings live closer to their parents than others, so the burden on those living closer is usually greater. If you are the one with the greater burden, it's only natural to get resentful and angry at the others, who are not carrying their share, who come to visit her less frequently—or not at all—who don't call that much—or not at all—and who, if called upon to kick in financially, drop the ball. Sure, you can get mad at them; then again, you might be one of them.

And what about your dad? How is he handling the situation? When I was in college, I would feel at times that Dad wasn't there enough for Mom. I thought that his playing golf, or finding another reason to go to the office rather than to a chemo session, was his way of skirting responsibility. I used to get mad at him. But I knew only peripherally what was really going on. The reality was that my mom didn't want my dad to come to her chemo sessions; they both were totally fine with that. I was just pushing my beliefs onto their situation, and that wasn't fair. This from a son who lived 1,500 miles away from them and saw them twice a year, at Christmas and in the summer. While I was going through law school, Mom and Dad were going through living hell, as my mom received chemo every week to stay alive.

Yet there I was, pointing my twenty-three-year-old finger at my dad, telling him that maybe he was shirking his job as a caregiver. Balls? Hardly. I was just trying to be protective of my mom, using my dad as the scapegoat. Such posturing, over time, only hurt my relationship with my dad, which took years to mend. I should have been more understanding and compassionate, but what I was really after was someone to take the blame for my mom's being so damn sick all the time. I took it out on a man who loved her more than anyone else, and who was hurting far worse than I knew at the time.

I didn't understand what my dad went through with his wife until I went through it with my own wife. It is important for a son, then, not to get in between parents when the mom is going through breast cancer. It simply is not your place, no matter how much you love and care for your mom, to tell your dad how to behave. The last thing that you need to do to your dad is make him feel that he has an enemy in you. It's their marriage, not yours, and you are always their child, not their marriage counselor.

Emotional Fallout as Her Father

It's always hard for men to relate to what a woman is going through with her body, but it is especially difficult for fathers. Many dads like to think of their daughters as women they must protect, and take care of, regardless of age. This innate protection mechanism often turns into a conflict with the daughter during her teenage years, and can get progressively worse as she goes off to college and enters adulthood. With cancer now in the picture, if she turns to you as her father for help, this doesn't mean that she has reverted to being a little girl. This is her disease, and it's her decision on how to treat it, not yours. At the same time, if the dad stays too removed from her condition, then she will perceive him as uncaring and not interested in her well-being.

Cindy, of Washington, D.C., had just finished an intense struggle with alcoholism before she was diagnosed with breast cancer. Her dad, living in Ohio, was involved with her alcohol problem, regularly calling her to see how she was doing and encouraging her to attend AA meetings on a regular basis. But when Cindy was diagnosed with breast cancer, he refused to visit her or speak with her on the phone. When she pressed her mom to put her dad on the phone, he refused. Why did he abandon her when she needed him most? Cindy's breast cancer had resurrected for her dad a family tragedy that happened years ago. Cindy's brother, Charles, was killed in a car accident while on his way to church, with her father at the wheel. The father lived and the son died, at age 16. Now that his daughter faced a life-threatening disease, it was too much for him to handle.

Another problem for dads, especially older ones, is the ability to talk about the emotional struggles that their daughters, and they, are going through. They would prefer to avoid the details and focus on just being present when needed. This approach can come across as cold, uncaring, and in some instances like abandonment.

Many daughters going through breast cancer have husbands, or boyfriends, and so friction can often arise between the men. The adage that "Father knows best" may come into play here. If the patient is married, the father must respect her marriage to another man and not intrude on that bond. Dads need to be respectful of the husband–wife relationship, no matter how troubled or difficult it appears to be from the outside. Dads must tread lightly around the husband, especially during the treatment process. He is the man of the house, not you. And unless you see either physical or emotional abuse, or excessive drinking or drug use, it is not your place to intervene. This is hard to do, especially if you are close to your daughter.

Another source of friction for fathers can occur if they have remarried, and there is a conflict between the new wife and the daughter. It is important for dad to show the daughter that she has the care and love of her father; he should not try to force love between a stepmother and daughter if it isn't there. This is especially true if the patient's mom—his ex—is involved in her care as well.

Dad must also be respectful about the amount of information the daughter feels comfortable sharing with him. He should not push too hard for details when not invited by his daughter to do so.

Emotional Fallout as Her Brother

The relationship between brothers and sisters, when they become adults, often suffers when there's distance between them. They often live in different cities, states, or parts of the world. But there is also the emotional distancing that happens as well. When siblings become adults, they may end up being very different people, with conflicting social, political, or religious approaches to life that cause them to not be as close as they once were.

Tensions that add to a brother–sister relationship may appear when she marries or becomes attached to someone that you, as her brother, don't particularly like or feel is good for her. Even if you have none of these problems with your sis (lucky for you), cancer has an incredible ability to get between you and her in ways you could never imagine. Given all that she has gone through, and continues to go through, she has been challenged in ways she probably has never been before. She is so vulnerable, especially in the later stages of her treatment, that any wrong thing you say, no matter how small or seemingly insignificant, could have a huge impact on how you continue to relate to her.

No matter how close you were to her before, the Big C monster often has an uncanny ability to get between you and your sister. For the record, it is easy for you to be the fall guy for her cancer troubles because often you are not around, especially if you live far away. If you had been close to her before, this may be the time of greater separation and alienation. She may not want you around; she might not want anyone around. For you, she will appear rundown, tired, and sickly, and this is going to get you down as well. And if, otherwise, your life is good, you might feel uncomfortable or guilty being happy around her.

With that said, as discussed earlier, you can be very instrumental in cheering her up through humor and pranks. But there are going to be times when she wants nothing to do with that. What then? Well, you must always take her lead and let things develop as she sees fit. Just being there for her is probably the best thing you can do, because it shows that you care. But if she wants time for herself, you have to respect that. Remember, too, that she may lash out at you and say hurtful things. This is a way for her, however messed up it is, to feel in command of those around her. Since she has lost control, for the moment, of her body because of the treatment, she might try to be controlling of you and the rest of her family and friends.

Having just gone through cancer treatment with my wife, I felt that when my sister Mary was diagnosed soon after, I would have all the right answers and the best things to say to her. Man, was I wrong. Each woman reacts differently to what she is going through. My sister, who is a very private person, just wanted to know that I was there for her, to comfort her, to listen to her, to be her big brother. I, meanwhile, felt that I could be of assistance in more ways than that because, after all, I had Sharon's experience fresh in my mind. The more I tried to push my view on my sister about what would be best for her, the more distant she became. Once she pointed this out to me, we were fine.

Emotional Fallout as Her Friend or Coworker

This is perhaps the hardest kind of caregiver to be, because most patients have families. However, she might want you to be the primary caregiver for the treatment, and not her family. Of course, you must always side with her and do whatever she wants. This may put you in a compromising position, so be very sensitive; don't get drawn into the middle of a mess between your loved one and her family. It is a no-man's-land, especially for you. When things go bad, you are going to be target number one. If you are a coworker, you have the added pressure of separating your work life from her personal life. After all, the last thing you want to do is put your job in jeopardy because you promised her to do things on the basis of her being an employee of the corporation.

. . . .
Mitigating the Emotional Fallout
. . . .

Now that you're in the thick of all that emotional fallout, how do you contain it? Whether you are a husband, son, father, brother, friend, or coworker, the radioactive fallout surrounds you. Treat this emotional radiation just as you would actual radiation. You have to suit up so you can put that contaminated material in a place where it can't continue to do any more damage. How and what you do to achieve this is different in each relationship, whether husband, son, father, brother, or friend/coworker. With breast cancer, silence is not golden; it's pure acid. You need to share your feelings with her and talk about what you are going through—and you need to do it as soon as you can. But how?

What worked for me was a technique called "dialoguing." It's a process by which participants become more aware of each other's needs, wants, and perceptions; basically, it helps people develop their communications abilities, which are founded on good listening skills. In dialoguing, there are four simple steps, which must be followed in order and without deviation:

Step 1. *Mirroring.* This begins with a simple statement by the speaker to the listener. When the speaker talks, he or she (because each person gets their chance to speak) expresses a thought in a short sentence that can be easily heard and understood by the listener. The listener then "mirrors" what the speaker just said, rephrasing it to confirm the meaning. If the speaker feels that the listener didn't hear what was said properly, then the speaker clarifies what was misunderstood. The listener then repeats the clarification. If the listener still hasn't gotten it right, he or she requests that the speaker use simpler sentences to help the listener better understand what is being said. It is crucial that the listener not add any comments or opinions about what the speaker has said. The listener then asks, "Is there more?" and there's more mirroring of the speaker's statements. It is very important that the listener only mirror what the speaker has said and nothing more.

Step 2. *Summarizing.* The listener repeats back to the speaker, in summary form, everything that the speaker has just said, in short concise sentences. If the listener has confused something that the speaker said, or the speaker feels the listener has gotten what the speaker said wrong, then the speaker needs to alert the listener regarding this. Once the clarification has been made, then the listener summarizes that mistake/clarification again until the speaker confirms that the listener has heard, and understood, everything correctly.

Step 3. *Empathy.* This is, without a doubt, the hardest and yet most vital step of the process. The listener must now identify one or more statements or points that the speaker has made, and then empathize with what that speaker has just said. By listening to what the speaker is saying, and understanding why he or she feels that way, the listener is now in a great position to empathize with the speaker—moving beyond the listener's own impressions and perceptions, by stepping into the speaker's shoes, so to speak. In this way, the listener is not only recognizing the validity of the speaker's perceptions, but also feeling, in a direct and empathetic way, all the speaker's feelings on a very personal level.

Step 4. *Switching Roles.* It's now time for the listener to speak, and the speaker to listen. This back-and-forth process should continue for as long as both the speaker and the listener feel comfortable dialoguing.

Getting to a place where you feel comfortable dialoging with your loved one may take a little while. For dialoguing to be successful, both she and you must follow its strict rules. If one person is really mad at the other, there may need to be a cooling-down period before you begin.

When I was so upset in Montreal, I certainly needed a cooling-down period before we could have discussed the problem through dialoguing. Indeed, I did literally cool down, in a pool. Montreal has one of the greatest pools in the world, built for the 1976 Olympics. I walked from a tiny locker room into the cavernous space with its soaring ceilings, several hundred feet high. The lanes were the widest lanes I have seen—it felt like I was swimming in my own river. Because the pool was so wide, the water barely moved as I swam my laps. Just hearing my regular breathing, over and over, calmed me. I realized that things really weren't as bad as I had built them up to be.

When I stepped out of the water, I was ready to rebuild my life with my wife. She was the most important thing in life. I returned to the hotel and saw Sharon lying on the bed, in tears. I was now ready to listen, and be heard, using the dialoguing process just described, and so was she. "Everything bad in our marriage had gotten worse because of cancer," Sharon said. "In the end, it was simply our love for each other that got us through it. It was extremely hard, but once we did get through, we were stronger than ever."

• • •

When life is overwhelming to you, go to a quiet room, be by yourself, and surrender to your feelings. Let them out; let those feelings wash over you. Listen to yourself, from deep inside. Also, stop the blame game. Blame doesn't help anyone, especially you—it's merely a cyclone that stirs up trouble and goes nowhere. Don't resent; instead, reset. Life is not about keeping score. There are no winners or losers when it comes to people you love. By hearing your true self speak, you will better understand what's going on inside, and you will be better able to explain to her what you've been feeling. In Montreal, I learned that my deepest fear was that my wife was going to die, just like my mom, and that feeling was what was coming between us.

If dialoging isn't the answer for you, then take advantage of the support resources available to caregivers, either from her treatment center or the various cancer organizations marked in the web resources section at the end of this book. These resources include psycho-oncologists, psychologists, and sociologists trained to deal with the mental health issues of breast cancer.

. . . .

Not All Radiation Is Bad

. . . .

Up until now, this chapter has been all about all the radioactive emotions that surround breast cancer. But radiation itself, in the medical sense, works wonders for survivability when it is part of the treatment regimen for your loved one.

Radiation oncology, also known as radiation therapy, targets the area or areas where her cancer had been found, and irradiates those areas to make sure the cancer never comes back again. It is also sometimes used as a first line of attack, when tumors are very large or have spread, to reduce them before surgery. The radiation regimen is usually five days a week for four to six weeks. Radiation does not hurt during the actual treatment, but there are a few side effects, the primary one being fatigue. Some others can include skin discoloration, redness, skin shrinkage, and wrinkling. More severe side effects include skin rupture or possible damage to important organs like the lungs or heart. Pregnant women cannot undergo radiation treatment until after delivery. The good news is that, as technology gets ever better, the risks become fewer. In particular, today's radiation oncology is able to pinpoint the targets much more effectively, which means that higher doses can be administered in shorter bursts. Shorter sessions also means the patient does not have to lie still for as long, allowing for more effective delivery of the radiation to the cancer regions.

The first visit to the radiology oncologist is to determine what the best treatment should be and to go through a trial run, or simulation, of the radiation. She may have marks (tattoos) placed on her chest, which are tiny blue or black dots used by the technician to locate the specific spot to radiate each time. The more the technician can make your loved one comfortable on the table, the better.

When my wife Sharon underwent radiation therapy, she was also in a clinical trial, taking Herceptin to treat her early stage cancer. At the time, doctors weren't sure what effect the drug would have on her heart, so she was constantly getting heart exams, or multiple gated acquisitions (MUGA) scans to make sure there was no damage to her heart tissue. The other unknown at the time was whether Herceptin, combined with radiation, could damage her heart in the long term. Studies that came out six years after Sharon's regimen confirmed she had made the right decision: there was no damage done by receiving simultaneous Herceptin and radiation treatments.

Sharon had radiation treatments five days a week for five weeks, plus five booster treatments to give her a "security blanket" of irradiation. That's a very long time, obviously; and over time it had a marked effect on her energy levels, making her very tired. The feeling of fatigue is cumulative, with more fatigue toward the end of the sessions than the beginning. There will be some days that are worse than others, especially if she has a booster treatment that gives an extra dose of radiation to the tumor area.

What does the caregiver offer during this time? You need to give her an extra boost emotionally. Appreciate everything that she has gone through to date and is continuing to face. Remember, one of the things she faces is her fears, because radiation therapy, especially before she gets her first treatment, "is something completely different and new, so many of them are scared," according to Dr. Randy Stevens, director of Radiation Oncology at White Plains Hospital. "Many [women] might know some bad stories from relatives or friends who were treated decades ago, with older radiation techniques. But for most women it is just something new, and that alone makes it scary. The anxiety [of radiation] might mean she could be terrified, that she might not be talking, that she might be angry and jumping down your throat when that is not normally her."

Once she begins the actual treatments, the radiation sessions are quick—an hour or less, including changing clothes or any other prep. It's a good idea for someone to be with her for the first appointment with the radiation oncologist, but after that she is usually fine on her own because she knows what to expect and can drive herself home.

For women getting radiation before chemo, or instead of chemo, the fatigue resulting from the treatments is apt to be a surprise. Dr. Stevens cautions, "so when they look great, their significant others often underestimate how tired they could really be. People expect them to be themselves. Some of my patients can be just as tired as chemo patients, but they don't look sick, so people don't rush to [help] them the way they do women who lose their hair." And the tiredness from radiation can last for months; recent studies have shown that recovery can take as long as a year to two. Keep this in mind, then, when you get impatient with your loved one because she is moving slowly or is not up for going out for a dinner party that night.

······················ CHAPTER 6 ······················

The New Normal

Rebuilding Her Life and Yours

· ·

FINALLY, IT'S OVER. After her last treatment, it's time to rebuild, reinvent, and reinvigorate her and your life again. The time has arrived when you leave Cancer Land and reenter daily life. Something has changed, however. The world she and you left when you went to Cancer Land no longer exists; instead, it has been transformed into the New Normal Life.

You thought that after treatment, you'd resume a regular, normal, everyday Joe kind of life, right? You've been craving, for so long, that "normal day"—starting with breakfast, the morning drive, work, and/or maybe a round of golf, tennis, the gym perhaps, lunch, dinner, TV viewing, then off to bed. Her doctors act like everything's back to the way it was as well. They no longer need to see your loved one all the time. She just has to check in with them every three or six months. But something is very different. She's different. She's a breast cancer survivor. As such, she no longer has her doctors, friends, and family hovering over her, but at the end of her day, she feels a deep sense of fear, even abandonment. She's facing what Penny Damaskos, coordinator of Memorial Sloan-Kettering Cancer Center's Post-Treatment Resource Program, calls a "point of crisis" moment.

Your loved one's first point of crisis happened back when she was diagnosed; her second was right before surgery. And now she faces her third, and arguably biggest, point of crisis: the time right after her treatment is over. Damaskos says that this is when patients feel that not only their medical team but also their personal support teams are no longer caring for her. Family members and others are saying, "This is great, you've finished with cancer," and they're all glad about it. She had been going to her doctors once or twice a week for months, and now they say they will see her in a couple of months. Suddenly, she feels that she alone has been left with the gigantic responsibility to be hypervigilant about cancer, watching the horizon to make sure nothing happens and it never shows its ugly face again. It's a weird, amorphous time when she begins to try and make sense of it all—"What happened?"

What *did* happen? This question leads many, if not most, breast cancer survivors into a heavy examination of their lives, now that survivorship is an integral part of who she is. Depending on your loved one, she may or may not want to make big changes in her life, while you just want to get back to the way things were before. "She is thinking that she is forever changed, and says to herself, 'I am not going back to the way things were,'" according to Damaskos. "Cancer has been a huge wake-up call to live her life differently."

So she asks herself: who am I after breast cancer? From this question comes perhaps an even greater one: what do I want to do with the rest of my life? This is when life-changing moments can occur. She may decide, for example, that she doesn't want to work anymore, or she wants to change careers, or she wants to travel more, or she wants to move to another part of the country, or she wants to change friends, or she wants to change partners, or she doesn't want to change anything until she knows what she wants. This is a time of great uncertainty, yet at the same time there is great hope for the future. It is a time to let her explore her new life. I encourage you to embrace her exploration of her future life as a breast cancer survivor. No matter what your relationship is with her—be it husband, father, son, brother, friend, boss, or coworker— you are facing a transition period during which you really don't know where the journey is going to end. But she is heading somewhere, off to her New Normal Life, as are you. So what is going to be her, and your, new story? What is that New Normal Life, and where does it begin?

. . . .

The New Medical Life

. . . .

Her and your views of the world have been changed. You don't see things in the same way any more. The petty matters of life aren't as important as they once were. You linger on things a little longer, show more patience, sit still longer. You enjoy being in the present. You can appreciate the simple stuff. "As is" is a good thing. Maybe this is what Lao-tzu, the ancient Chinese philosopher, was thinking when he jotted down this little mental nugget: "The way to do is to be."

Fresh things taste fresher. There is a bit more crispness to the air, sharpness in the sky. That's because she's taken her first step forward—cancer free! Your loved one's breast cancer, until proven otherwise, has been defeated. That's not to say that the fear of its coming back has gone away. But her doctors believe that her cancer is gone; her family, friends, and coworkers believe it is gone; and so you and she must begin believing that, too. Until she gets over this fear of its coming back, she will live as if she were still in her old medical reality—a breast cancer patient. No, she needs to be in her new medical reality as a breast cancer survivor, who will fight and protect her body from cancer ever invading again.

There is an old saying about the three Rs that a student in elementary school must learn to be successful in life: reading, w(r)iting, and a(r)ithmetic. Likewise, there are three Rs that she must learn in her new medical reality, too: reexamining, restoring, and rejuvenating her life after breast cancer.

Reexamining

The best thing that your loved one can do for herself is to have regular checkups with her breast cancer medical team. Her checkup requirements will vary depending on her initial cancer diagnosis, but the norm is a visit every three months for the first few years, with follow-up appointments every six months after that, when she gets the necessary scans and blood work.

She needs to make sure that she is receiving the latest and greatest medical care. Every year, the diagnostic tools get better, the surgical procedures get more accurate, the medicines get more effective, and the radiation therapies more thorough. So your loved one will want to keep up with the latest medical innovations. If she finds that her doctors are no longer following the best medical procedures, then she should consider looking elsewhere. For example, it doesn't hurt to get a second opinion after treatment as well. After we moved from New York to Virginia, Sharon signed on with a new oncologist, but also kept her regular oncologist in New York, Dr. Bonnie Reichman, based on the theory that two heads are better than one.

With this said, many women are not as vigilant as they should be after treatment ends. Researchers at the University of Massachusetts Medical School found in a study of over 800 breast cancer survivors over the age of fifty-five that 80 percent of these women were screened the first year after ending treatment, but only 63 percent were by the fifth year. Perhaps the most alarming statistic in this study was that only *one-third* of the women studied got an annual mammogram, despite the fact that all of them had health insurance, had full access to mammography centers, and, most important, had a three times higher risk of recurrence than women who never had cancer.

Why? Denial is still a very powerful emotion. You might hear your loved one say, "What I don't know, won't hurt me." BS, right? So it's your job to make extra sure that your loved one continues to get her regularly scheduled checkups *and* an annual mammogram.

Reexamining also includes what she can do to lead a more healthful life. A great place to start is diet, especially a low-fat, high-vegetable/fruit diet. But she shouldn't stop there. Regular exercise is a great way to build her immune system. If she adds weight lifting or weight-bearing exercises to the mix, that will help prevent bone loss, which she may be suffering from as a side effect of hormonal drugs that she's taking. Another great immune builder is sleep. If she's a smoker, she should stop; studies have shown that smoking lowers the immune system, as well as possibly stimulating residual cancer cells in the body.

Despite her best intentions to lead a healthier life, of course, you cannot mandate these changes because, that's right, it's her body, not yours. You can make suggestions, but you can't force her to follow them. The key here is to accept her, and love her for how she wants to live her life. I had a hard time with this when it came to my wife during her first year of posttreatment. She was suffering from early stages of osteoporosis because of the drugs she was taking, as well as a loss of energy, and it was killing me that she refused to get regular exercise. So I challenged her to change, and we fought about it, a lot—to the detriment of our relationship. I thought that I was acting out of love, as her husband, trying to get her to do what was best for her body. She, meanwhile, felt that I was overstepping my bounds (she was right, as she almost always is).

The reexamination of medical life doesn't stop with her; it's time for you to reexamine your medical life as well. It's no surprise that caregivers of breast cancer patients suffer physically during the process. In most cases, they have abandoned their exercise regimens, eaten poorly, slept badly, perhaps been drinking or smoking a bit too much, and suffered through inordinate amounts of stress and depression. This is bad news for you, so something must be changed in your new life also. You must now eat right and drink responsibly, for your own good. The last thing that she needs is for something bad to happen to you, after all that she has just been through.

I know that my immune system was crushed when I went through not one but two breast cancer experiences, first with my wife and then with my sister. I felt tired all the time, and achy all over. When I would drive Sharon to her chemo and radiation appointments, my left knee would start to hurt. Of course, like most guys, I didn't do anything about it until my wife bugged me incessantly to see the doctor. It turned out there was something wrong with me: I had Lyme disease, which I had contracted from a deer tick bite, probably from when I would run through the woods near my house in Westchester County, New York. But my medical condition didn't stop there. I had been coughing more than usual, so my doctor ordered some chest X-rays to make sure that I didn't have pneumonia. I didn't, but I did test positive for tuberculosis.

I must have been exposed to some homeless fellow on the subway while riding to work in New York City. It turned out that the TB was "walled," so it wasn't active. But it was there, nonetheless. When I came home to tell Sharon that I had tested positive for not only Lyme disease but also tuberculosis, she started laughing. "I always thought of you as competitive, but I never thought you'd be so competitive as to compete with me in diseases," she said.

I went on a regimen of doxycycline for the Lyme and X-ray monitoring for the TB over the next year, and all my symptoms and concerns went away. My wife and sister, meanwhile, began their regimens of hormonal drugs to make sure their cancer never came back. But their preventive medical actions didn't stop there.

A breast cancer survivor may have a greater risk of ovarian cancer. If she does, then getting a hysterectomy or removal of her ovaries and fallopian tubes may be recommended by her medical team. This is a personal decision because this procedure, like the breast cancer treatment that preceded it, hits dead center at her femininity. In deciding whether to have a hysterectomy or not, she must consider not only the risks of contracting ovarian cancer but also whether she wants to have children.

My sister decided to do genetic testing to find out if she carried mutations in the breast cancer genes, BRCA1 or BRCA2. When the tests came back that she was, in fact, a BRCA2 mutation carrier, she realized that placed her at a much higher risk of contracting ovarian or fallopian cancer later in life. So she opted for a complete hysterectomy to remove all worries on that front, even though some doctors said that removal of her ovaries and fallopian tubes would have been enough. Sharon had the same surgery performed because of the extreme aggressiveness of her breast cancer.

They both felt comfortable moving forward with this operation because they didn't want any more children. But what if your loved one hasn't had any children yet—or wants another after she's been treated? That's right; it's her decision. But the key thing for you is to make sure that, if she decides to move forward to have a child after breast cancer, it is an informed decision. It's no secret that having a baby stimulates estrogen production, which can be fertile ground for cancer cells.

If she wants to have a baby, an important addition to her medical team is her gynecologist, and perhaps a fertility specialist as well. The best time for women of childbearing age to talk with a fertility specialist and her oncologist about having a baby is ideally before chemotherapy ever begins (assuming she is having chemotherapy treatment) so that proper coordination can be made between her oncologist/gynecologist/fertility expert team.

If she didn't have the talk about having a baby before treatment and now wants a baby, the sooner she has that discussion with her doctors the better. The first question to ask, before all others, is whether she is able to have a baby. If she has received chemotherapy, she may already have undergone early menopause. This is when a fertility expert comes in handy. If she does want a baby, it's a balancing act to make sure that she doesn't go into early menopause *and* that her estrogen levels aren't so high as to promote the return of cancer.

Preventing a new cancer in the opposite breast may include a prophylactic mastectomy, if she is a gene carrier that puts her at high risk for cancer to appear in that breast. As if that is not enough to worry or think about, there is the possibility that she could get other cancers, not related to her original breast cancer. My mom, in between her breast cancer recurrences, was diagnosed with colon cancer, as was my dad. I attribute this to a low-fiber diet, which my mom was forced to cook for the large family on a tight budget, providing a feed trough of spaghetti, mac and cheese, and Chef Boyardee pizzas smothered in Bacos; but the real reason was probably more related to genetics. Since today's genetic testing methods were not available back then, I'll never really know.

Speaking of medical care, what have you done to make sure that you stay healthy? When was your last medical checkup? Have you kept up with age-appropriate tests for prostate and colon cancer? If you are fifty or older, for example, you should schedule a colonoscopy and sign up for a PSA test done to check your prostate (even though interim findings from a study by the National Cancer Institute this year show no evidence of a survival benefit, raising the question of whether the test leads to overdiagnosis and overtreatment for prostate cancer). If breast cancer teaches us anything, it is that life is precious and must be protected by drawing upon the best that the medical profession has to offer.

Men are notorious for not taking care of themselves. They don't go to doctors when they have symptoms, and often they wait until the symptoms turn into a condition. Perhaps that's the number one reason we don't live as long as women. I remember when my granddaddy pooh-poohed the significance of doctors. He was a farmer, and he thought that if you ate right, exercised, and slept well, you'd lead a long life. Since he was well into his seventies, he used his own life as the poster child example for his life philosophy. All was well, that is, until he started feeling a nagging pain in his side, which never seemed to go away. When he started to see blood in his stool, he thought that maybe it was finally time to visit the doc. He found out that he had prostate cancer, and that if he had gone to the doctor when he first got the symptoms, he would have been fine. But he didn't, and so the cancer had spread throughout his body, finally showing up in his colon, which caused the bleeding.

With the cancer now in his liver as well, he was terminal, with no future hope of survival. He made me promise that I would never let that happen to me. It was sad because at the time I was just starting to date Sharon, whom I would later see through cancer as well. He was a proud man and didn't want to meet her in his compromised sick state. Nevertheless, I often think how valuable that meeting would have been for my wife, now that she has faced cancer herself.

So when was your last physical? You can't attack a medical problem that you *might* have until you know you have it. Preventative screenings for cancers, done early, can catch it before it catches you, like it did to my beloved granddaddy.

There is a growing movement afoot in the United States to focus more on preventive care than reactive care. By attacking health conditions before they become chronic or terminal, we will see more people lead happier, healthier lives. It's the apple a day keeps the doctor away approach to living. Insurance companies are catching on to this concept as well. I signed up for a policy that covers annual physicals, flu shots, and lower fees for routine doctor visits. Previously, my family had an old-fashioned policy that had a higher copay for regular visits to a doctor. So, what usually happens when you have to pay more for routine physician visits out of pocket? You put off going to the doctor. For example, I put off going for this annoying knee ailment that never seemed to go away, which, as I mentioned earlier, turned out to be Lyme disease. I never got that telltale red circular rash that is characteristic of early stage Lyme. Finally, after a few months delay, I went, and it's a good thing that I did because my condition would have continued to deteriorate, going from a gimpy walk to possible facial paralysis, advanced arthritis, hand and feet numbness, fevers, and possibly brain swelling, leading to meningitis and memory loss.

It's not a bad idea to undergo a genetic test to see if you are carrying a deleterious or disease-related mutation in BRCA 1 or 2. We all have these genes, but if you have inherited a mutation in one copy of one of the genes that is linked to disease causation, then you and your close relatives are at much higher risk for early-onset breast cancer, bilateral breast cancer and ovarian cancer. If many individuals in your family history have had breast and or ovarian cancer or early-onset cancer, or if you know that other family members carry mutations in either gene, you might consider genetic counseling and testing. If you are related to someone who has a BRCA 1 or BRCA 2 mutation, you might also have inherited the mutation, and then have a higher risk of breast and/or ovarian cancer (that's right, men get breast cancer, too), or other forms of cancer like prostate, pancreatic, or colon cancer. If you are the husband and you and your wife have children, the gene can be passed on to your kids. That means if you have daughters, they will have a higher statistical chance of getting breast cancer and so will need to be closely monitored. My dad got tested, and he found out that he carried a mutated or abnormal form of the BRCA1 gene. My sister and I have had only boys, but any daughters that my brothers have, or my sons, might carry a high risk of contracting breast cancer in their lifetimes if they inherit the mutated gene.

Restoring

Her body has been through a tremendous battle, and now that the battle is over, she needs to begin restoring her body in the best way that she can. This starts with eating right, and means that she should include more fruits, vegetables, and other cancer-fighting foods in her meals and snacks to strengthen her immune system. Check if her insurance company will pay for a consultation with a nutritionist; if not, look into the possibility of paying for a private consultation instead. It's well worth the money to get started again on the right nutritional track.

It would be great to encourage her to begin an exercise program. A side effect of many of the drugs is bone density loss. A simple and easy way to help counter osteoporosis is weight training. Studies have shown that lifting is a great way for women to slow the loss of bone density. There are an infinite number of exercise programs from which she can choose, so she should pick the one that she will enjoy the most. It could be yoga, walking, weight training, swimming, hiking, kickboxing, boxing, biking, and anything in between.

A part of the program to stop or slow bone loss is for her to take a calcium supplement every day with meals and take the appropriate vitamin D as prescribed by her doctor. Since there are all kinds of supplements on the shelves today, doctors usually recommend that she use one that allows high absorption into her body. The daily recommended calcium levels vary depending on her age. Calcium is absorbed through the small intestine. To help this absorption, vitamin D is added to the calcium supplement. Also, the more acidic her small intestine is, the better the absorption of calcium. So the most efficient calcium absorption is through a calcium citrate pill.

Since your body is battle-fatigued as well, consider what your own exercise and supplement regime will be now. You probably have been feeling worn down, tired, and, yes, depressed. You need to jump-start your own physical care. Start with a set of tennis or two, or a walk around the block—anything to get you active and out of the house.

Rejuvenating

This is the last step in the new medical process. If she has had chemotherapy, this could be when she gets all of her hair back. Sometimes, her hair will come back in a different shade, possibly even a different color altogether. Her hair's texture could also be different. She may well prefer that new shade or texture (certainly you would hope so).

Her body may have changed as well. In addition to the operation or operations on her breasts, her weight may have gone up or down. Her energy level may be different. As mentioned earlier, her sexual energy and interest may well have changed. So when we talk about rejuvenation, we are looking to help her find the new her, not the same person she was before cancer. You must embrace and accept those differences. Rejuvenation is not about going back to the way it was; it's about moving forward to the new. Rejuvenation means "to make young again," but in the Stand by Her world, it is about invigorating her passion and vitality, rekindling her inner fire, and renewing her zest for life.

Your own rejuvenation is also at hand. Caregiving is hard work, and you've been through a lot, so the last thing you're probably thinking about is taking care of yourself. Well, do it. Right after Sharon finished her last treatment, I went on a golf trip with my dad and my brothers. They did everything they could to get my mind off of cancer. I was surrounded by people who wanted to take care of me. If golf isn't your thing, maybe it's a card game, or tennis, or a reading club. Get back to who you are.

················
The New Emotional Life
················

After treatment, she might become depressed. It's probably not something you'd expect, but it does happen. Consider this: from the time she got her first diagnosis, she has been in "queen warrior" mode; now, her fight is over, and the battle has been won—or has it? Certainly it has been won in a physical sense, but the emotional struggle often begins now, after treatment. The struggle has been put on hold, and now she must face the problems and fears head-on.

So, she may have to go back to dealing with problems in her marriage, or with her family or friends, that existed before cancer came into her life. She also may feel abandonment. Her doctors are not hovering over her any longer, and neither are her family and friends. This leaves her to herself, alone, to decide who she is and who she wants to be for the rest of her life. She's just had a huge wake-up call.

This, then, requires a period of reflection, not only for her but for you as well.

Reflecting

Reflection is looking at life in a detached and comprehensive manner. Our society discourages us from reflecting on where we are and where we want to be, as well as who we are. We are, instead, pushed to *do* things, to "get 'er done." The quicker the better.

But it's time to set down our BlackBerries and iPods and process what we have just been through. Consider taking some time off from work (assuming that you haven't used up all your time already) and going somewhere, away from the world's distractions. Some folks prefer the mountains, others the beach, still others the desert. It could be a spa or a state park. Wherever the setting, set some time alone to look at yourself, and your loved one. See all the things about your lives that have changed owing to the cancer, both positive and negative, and just let those observations settle in for a while. Think of them as drifting wood on a calm lake, just floating by for observation.

That calm water is the inner you. It is a reflection of your past. But when you peer closer, into the water itself, you see the new you—what you've become. True reflection is not done in a minute, an hour, or even a day. No, true reflection happens over time, because you are processing experiences that at first appear jumbled, jagged, and unconnected. Reflection allows you to begin to see how all these experiences make sense. Consider writing down your thoughts, in a notebook, journal, or just on random sheets of paper.

After a few weeks or a month later, review what you wrote. You'll still be reflecting and assessing, but you'll begin to identify, among all those deep thoughts, your distractions, your impulsive raw feelings, and your reactions to what has happened to you in Cancer Land.

Reacting

How many stories have we read about soldiers, returning from war, who have incredible difficulty readjusting to civilian life? They can't concentrate. They can't keep a job. They have difficulty communicating. They can't function properly. That's because they are suffering from post-traumatic stress disorder (PTSD), which is defined by the National Institute of Mental Health (NIMH) as an "anxiety disorder that can develop after exposure to a terrifying event or ordeal in which grave physical harm occurred or was threatened." Certainly your loved one faced grave physical harm, and you faced it as well by association. The NIMH says, "People with PTSD have persistent frightening thoughts and memories of their ordeal and feel emotionally numb, especially with people they were once close to. They may

experience sleep problems, feel detached or numb, or be easily startled."

The hardest part about the posttreatment phase, for patients
and caregivers alike, is changing from the mind-set that both of you
needed to fight the cancer war. You feel like a warrior who has just
put away his weapons—but you're not sure if the war is truly over
yet, and that brings a lot of anxiety. This happens right when everyone else around you is saying, "You must be so happy to be done
with cancer." And this is where reactions come flooding into your
world. You might get mad at your loved one, or others, for no understandable reason. You might find yourself unable to sleep at
night, mindlessly clicking the cable channels. You might have attention problems at work or at home with your family. You might just
feel down and can't figure out why. You might feel blah—that nothing really matters any more.

You are having Cancer Land withdrawal. You'd think that this
is the last place you would end up—and it is. But for the past year,
or longer, you have only known Cancer Land, and now you are back
in the real world—where no one seems to care and certainly where
no one understands.

As far as your loved one goes, she is having reactions to her
cancer as well. Some of these reactions might be mild and others
might be extreme. For example, she may want to quit her job, move
to another city, go back to school. One breast cancer survivor decided that the reason she made it through her treatments was because of fairies, so, in tribute to the little winged creatures, she built
houses in the woods for her newfound supernatural friends; that way,
she could visit them on a daily basis, at the base of oak trees, in little
stone huts, and in tiny wooden structures along a nearby creek. She
had left the real world for Neverland.

Thankfully, this is an extreme example of where breast cancer
survivors can go in posttreatment. Nonetheless, it is normal for her
to have reactions during this new chapter of her life. Some of these
reactions can be wonderful, and profound. My wife, for example,
committed her newfound life to becoming a breast cancer advocate,
volunteering to speak with other women recently diagnosed and be-

coming a legislative advocate at both state and federal levels for the Susan G. Komen for the Cure. My sister went back to work as a nurse, but instead of working at a hospital, she switched to hospice care, helping terminal cancer patients. My mom turned her energies to kids, working as a nurse at a preschool, being the team mom for my sister's cross-country team, and being on the school board of my brothers' high school.

Some women change their careers, though not always because they wanted to. Dawn, of South Carolina, could no longer be a speech pathologist for young children because of her compromised immune system after the chemo, so she worked with adults instead. For some women, their work no longer has as much meaning, so they change from full-time to part-time employment, or leave the workforce altogether. The latter, of course, can put a stress on the marriage, especially in tough economic times, so encourage her to talk this over with her husband before she acts on impulse.

Resolving

This step is the culmination of reflection and reaction, the step in which they merge like yin and yang to formulate an emotional whole. If true resolution takes place, life becomes simpler, calmer, better. Every step in this new life has meaning and significance that makes sense of what once seemed like random events. Resolution gives purpose to life. You have a wish list, and you keep the promises you make to yourself. When, and if, this happens, you do what you truly want to do, you participate in activities that have meaning for you, you spend time with people you really care about, and ideally you find true joy in your day-to-day life.

. . . .

The New Financial Life

. . . .

With the recent economic turmoil, more and more breast cancer patients are facing bills that they won't be able to pay—right away, if at all. So how can she navigate the blizzard of medical debts that swirl around her after treatment, and what can you do to help her get through this financial storm?

Reimbursing (and Paying)

The first thing she needs to do is get her doctor and hospital bills paid. Depending on her work, finances, or age, payments could come from the insurance company, the military, Medicare, Medicaid, her family and friends, or her own pocket. The key to bill payment is to line up the bills and make sure that the proper processing has begun, and that someone stays on top of it. It's so easy to get confused by medical bills. They are long and detailed, and contain similar-sounding language. So, separate the bills according to the stage in the treatment process; for example, have separate piles for diagnosis, surgery, chemo, and radiation. Check them for accuracy, as mistakes are frequently made.

If she has insurance coverage, she should make sure that all her bills are processed through her carrier. Once the bills have been processed, she or someone she appoints, should double-check the math to ascertain that the carrier is paying the bills in accordance with the policy terms, and that any payments owed by her as a deductible or copay are accurate. Insurance companies usually send what is known as an "explanation of benefits," which breaks down the deductibles and copays owed by the patient and the percentages paid, and owed, by the insurer and patient, respectively. The bills need to match the insurer's explanation of benefits; if they don't, then work out the discrepancies between the doctor's billing department and the carrier.

As discussed earlier in the book, she should have gotten all medical procedures for her treatment preauthorized so that the insurer pays the bills owed her doctors. Sometimes the preauthorization falls through the cracks; if it does, get the carrier to recognize that a preauthorization had been made. She should lean on her doctor's billing department to get this situation fixed as soon as possible, to make that problem go away. If any claim is denied by her insurance, she should appeal it. If the company then denies her appeal, she should demand an in-person hearing. If this hearing goes against her, she's still not done: she can contact the state's department of insurance to file a claim against the insurance company.

If your loved one's insurance is through an employer, she can get her human resources department involved in processing the claim. A final option is to hire a lawyer and file a claim against the insurance company for her day in court. If her insurance policy is obtuse, unclear, and downright misleading, a judge may rule against the company and force it to cover part, or possibly all, of the charges involved.

One last thing. Her medical payments, if more than 5 percent of her income, may be deductible on her income tax return. Check with an accountant or the IRS for more details.

Recovering

The cancer wars can leave survivors financially drained. If she works, and had to either cut back or abandon her job, she may face serious debts. If you are her husband, you may be equally responsible for these debts so you could ask for a raise, if it is the right time to do so. Just don't use your wife's cancer as the reason; her illness has nothing to do with your performance on the job and your value to the company. Consider, however, if you haven't asked for a raise in quite some time, your situation could be an incentive to get paid what you deserve. If a raise is not possible, think about taking a second job or starting a side business. Now that she is back to normal, she can also seek work if she doesn't have a job already or perhaps ask for a raise as well if she does.

If she is in serious financial straits, and money is needed immediately, one approach is to borrow money from family and friends. This is a tough thing for many folks to do, however, because of the emotional baggage that accompanies such requests. She should do what feels comfortable—for borrowed money in family situations can turn very ugly, indeed. A much better option might be to see if she qualifies for either state or federal assistance. The key here is to respect what she is most comfortable doing, and don't talk her into taking money that she may later regret.

Another option is to pay the bills by credit card or take out a home equity line of credit. The problem with credit card payments is the added cost of interest, often set at high percentages. As for the home equity approach, this carries with it the risk that, if she doesn't pay back the money she's borrowed, then she could lose her home through foreclosure. Also, she may not have this option if housing values have dropped and her mortgage is higher than the equity she has in her house.

Finally, if she can't afford to pay the bill, she can ask the various medical providers to adjust the amounts owed or work out a long-term payment plan.

Replenishing

The goal is for your loved one to get back to where she was financially before she was diagnosed. This might take months or years to achieve, however, as cancer is costly. If she is not working or is retired, then full replenishment might not be possible. To fill in the difference, she might apply for assistance from government agencies, such as Social Security, Medicare, or Medicaid. If she is working, then maybe she can better her income by going back to school and studying for a new career with a higher earning potential.

After a diagnosis of cancer, it's more difficult to think in the long term. Nevertheless, everyone is responsible for his or her retirement, so her financial considerations must include future plans, and that involves savings as well. To make this possible, she must be prepared to tighten her belt—to budget household expenses carefully. It could be as simple as collecting coupons, or cutting out a vacation, restaurants, new clothing, or not buying that new car right away. Or it could involve a more severe lifestyle change for her, depending on her situation.

. . . .

The New Married Life

. . . .

Many husbands, like I did, think that when her treatment is over the marriage will go right back to the way it was before she got cancer. But, as we know, that isn't going to happen. You can't go back the way you came; that door is closed, forever. One of the reasons you can't go back is that feeling of loss she has. She has faced, for months now, a loss of her femininity, and if she has had a mastectomy, she has also suffered a devastating loss of her breast or breasts. So the best thing that you can do for both of you is to rekindle the marital fire.

Rekindling

Think of your romantic life as starting all over again. As you did when you first met her, make her feel special. This must be done carefully, gently, and very slowly, of course. Just as you use small sticks and saplings to start a real fire, use small and simple gestures to refire your marriage.

Remember how, when you first laid eyes on her, you wanted to ask her out? Well, ask her out again. Seriously—ask her out on a date. Tap into those romantic feelings that first brought the two of you together. The difference is that, now, the "new" woman you are attracted to is your "new" wife, whom you love more than ever. Your focus is on looking forward, not back. You need to show her that you still care for her, are still attracted to her, still want her, just the way she is—now.

It's normal if she has been feeling alone, because she probably is the only woman in her immediate circle who has just gone through this traumatic experience. So, to make her feel part of you, embrace her. Start slowly, and show her how much you love her by touching her, holding her, caressing her. Next, show your romantic side—that you have been thinking of her, and do something that will make her feel special.

This doesn't mean that you have to spend a lot of money on her. Simple, thoughtful things, in fact, work best. Write her a note, telling her how proud you are to be her husband. Take her to her favorite restaurant and make a big fuss over how great she looks. Take a walk with her, or watch a movie that she wants to see. The key is to spend quality time with her, and get comfortable with each other again. Keep in mind that both of you have been changed by this experience—and you both will probably realize that both of you have changed. You are different people, and it takes time to find out who you are—and that involves revelation.

Revealing

A lot of feelings were shelved when she got breast cancer. A lot of things were not said between the two of you during her treatment. After all, there was the cancer to think about. It was not just part of the world, it was your whole world. Now that "it" is no longer in her, no longer part of your life, it is time to figure out what is in your life. Given the amount of change that has occurred, this isn't going to be that easy to do! You must first discover what new land she and you now inhabit.

It's almost as if you were lost at sea and landed on an uncharted island as the only two survivors. You have to explore the terrain. You will be disoriented, and so you must express your thoughts and feelings in an open and honest way. This may not come naturally for you. One approach is to use the dialoging method, detailed in the last chapter: it forces each of you to listen and really comprehend what the other is saying, and more important, feeling. You have to know you are being heard, and so does she, as well as being understood.

You might not know, initially, what your true feelings are. So much in your life has been rearranged, even ravaged, that it is hard to know what to order at a diner for breakfast, let alone expose your inner feelings to your loved one. So you must be patient.

Start the process and reveal your feelings first. So much attention has been placed on your loved one that it will probably be a relief for her to have you take center stage for awhile. With that said, be aware of what she has gone through, and continues to go through, when you open up. You don't want her to feel that she is now somehow inadequate.

Don't be surprised if she has a ton of revealing to do as well. She may want to share some things about you that aren't going to be pleasant to hear. You need to accept that, for this process is about getting things out into the open, so you can discuss them, analyze them, and resolve these issues. At times, it might seem that your talks are more like peace negotiations. But when things get a bit heated, rely on the love and respect you have for each other and let those foundations lead the way through this difficult time.

I failed to follow my own advice here, and it nearly cost me my marriage. I had put a lot of personal problems on hold during Sharon's cancer treatment; these were feelings I either wasn't being honest about or, in other instances, was too forceful about. It got so bad between us, in fact, that I had to leave the house for a while. This drastic action jump-started us to the negotiating table to work things out. The one thing that we had going for us—the most important thing—was our love for each other.

The most difficult time for us happened on Thanksgiving Day. Sharon and I both felt that our marriage was coming apart, and, for the first time, had a real possibility of ending. We had been invited to a party at a swanky apartment on New York City's Upper West Side, which had a bird's-eye view of the Macy's Day Parade. All I wanted to do was reach out, jump on top of Big Bird or Pikachu, and float away on a helium airship, escaping the marital turmoil forever. But I also wanted our marriage to make it, and I was willing to do the work. I needed to be open with her, vulnerable to her—to be myself. It was clear that we needed someone else to help knock down the blockade between us.

We turned to a marriage counselor, Lisa Baroni, who in her words helped us "reknit" our marriage. "This cancer had stepped in and really wrecked havoc," according to Baroni. "It attacked the family. It attacked the relationship. This is not a couple who would have presented [to me for counseling] if cancer hadn't happened."

Sharon and I walked up several flights of stairs each week to meet with Baroni in the garret of an old stone Episcopal Church in Armonk, New York. The place had a holy vibe about it, in no small part because it was in a historic church, which I think had a subconscious effect on us about the sanctity of marriage, which was a good thing. The big issue that emerged during these sessions was my fear of Sharon's dying from cancer, because cancer had stolen my mom from me. When this fear was brought out into the open, Sharon "was able to offer incredible empathy and support. She was so sad and upset because John was so sad and upset," according to Baroni. "I looked at this couple, thinking 'wow, they are reknitting themselves back together by talking about how scary it is to consider losing somebody—while at the same time losing their lives before cancer.'" In other words, we still loved each other very much. Thanks to those therapy sessions, we were able to pass through our period of marital darkness and reach the light. We had followed The Doors' Jim Morrison's mantra—"Break on Through (To the Other Side)."

Marriage counseling saved us. There are so many problems that surface between a husband and wife after cancer treatment— problems with regard to the marriage, not the cancer. When these preexisting conditions resurface in this new life, they come up raw, sudden, and without filtration because cancer has stripped away the couple's coping mechanisms. So I strongly recommend that all couples, whatever their marital stability, book a routine visit with a local marital counselor, if for no other reason than to get a tune-up for their relationship and unclog any channels of communication *before* problems arise. You don't want a situation where, "the husband and wife talk to each other with tacks spitting out of their mouths," according to Baroni. We take our cars in for repairs, we hire handymen to fix our houses, but we hesitate to get help with our marriages until it is too late. What's wrong with having marital maintenance work done once in a while? Nothing. Nothing at all.

Renewing

You've probably been to at least one renewal ceremony, at which a married couple renews their vows before their family and friends. It's a celebration, a special wedding anniversary. But what is the purpose of this ceremony? After all, they are already married. Well, it is a romantic reboot, a renewed commitment made before the world that this husband and wife still love each other so much that they are willing to proclaim that love in a formal public setting, again. It says that, after all the ups and downs, positives and negatives, changes and stases in their marriage, they still love each other enough to celebrate their oneness, to have and to hold, together, until death.

A lot changes between couples after they are married. They not only look differently, they think differently, act differently, pray differently, work differently, believe differently from how they did before marriage or in the first couple of years of marriage. I know that's true with me. I am turning fifty this year, and I certainly am not the same man that I was when I walked down the aisle at the age of thirty-two with Sharon. The biggest change is the loss of innocence and naiveté that I had back then. But what I gained in its place was wisdom, patience, and understanding. A lot has changed with my wife too—all for the better, of course.

If ever there is a time for a renewal between a husband and wife it is after breast cancer. This is when you renew your commitment to each other, when the two of you not only embrace the tremendous changes that have happened because of this disease, but also proclaim to the world that cancer has brought you closer together than you've ever been before. The renewal is a spiritual thing. Your loved one and you have been dragged through the sludge, to emerge from the mud better than ever before. You have become more grounded, practical, and aware of the world. These sensations may not be immediate, like a bright-light epiphany, but in the end you are left with a fuzzy, warm feeling and assurances of security, sanity, and satisfaction. It's no longer about past or future wants and regrets. It's about acceptance, absolution, and embracing each other in the present moment.

. . . .

The New Father and Daughter Life

. . . .

There is perhaps no more protective relationship in humanity than that of a father to his daughter. This instinct was heightened when she was diagnosed, which threatened the life of your precious little girl. And now, here you are, being told that this threat is over and that it's time for you to let her go. This isn't going to be easy to do. During these past months, she may have been clutching you for security, for guidance, for comfort—and now it's time for her to leave you and get back to her regular life.

She may have been living in your house, and now she is ready to go home. She may have made you her closest confidant when things got rough with her husband or boyfriend; now that she's better, now that she's a survivor, it's time to let her go again. The first time she left you to go off into the big world was hard enough. This time it might be even harder, because the last thing that you want is for your daughter to get sick again. You are torn up inside, asking yourself over and over again, is she going to be all right?

Releasing

There is that old adage every father has heard at some point in his parenthood: father knows best. It comes from that 1950s show of the same name, in which Jim Anderson, the father, is an insurance agent who raises three children—Betty, Bud, and Kathy. He's a man of the world, with all the wisdom in the world to impart to his family, because, after all, he knew best—about everything. He was the fella who sat by the fire in his cardigan sweater, walked the dog, and had a regular nine to five gig at work. Well, that Pop is long gone. As we all know, but especially during cancer, your daughter may have turned to you for advice and comfort in ways that reminded you of the relationship you had with her when she was young. Now that her treatment is over, it's time to release her back into the real world.

The best way to let her go is to provide positive reinforcement about how proud of her you are, and will continue to be, now that she's a breast cancer survivor. Whatever she decides to do after treatment needs to be fine by you. She is reestablishing her new normal life, so the last thing that she needs right now is disapproval from her dear old dad. She is an adult, and so it is critical that you respect her opinions and decisions. It's time to give her a big hug, and let her go.

Reassuring

It is important for you, posttreatment, to periodically check in with your daughter to see how she's doing. Don't presume that everything is back to normal. Your daughter, for the next few years at least, is going to be continually worried that her cancer might come back. She needs your reassurance that everything is going to be fine, that all is well again in the world. Let her know that you love her, and care.

My dad has made a point of calling my sister every week or so, just to see how she is doing and to let her know that he is thinking about her. My father-in-law, who lives in our town, takes my wife out every week to lunch just so he can check in with her, see how she's doing, and have some great one-on-one time with his only daughter. Additionally, we have a family dinner with him, his wife Mary, and our kids every Sunday night, as well. He makes himself available to Sharon whenever she needs to talk. I'm not saying all fathers have to do all this, but I am saying to just be vigilant in keeping open the channels of communication with your daughter, achieved by listening to her on an ongoing basis.

If your daughter is single, she may be having problems with her body image and may be fearful that she will never find a mate. Continually pay her compliments on the way she looks. Be sincere when you make these compliments, because if she doesn't believe you, then you will do more harm than good to her self-esteem.

Returning

When a dad follows up with his daughter, it shows her that he cares. If you're a dad who lives in another town or state, get back to see her again as soon as you can. Physically being there for her is a testament of your love for her. And when you are with her, her family, and friends, be the listener and not the speaker. Your role is all about making her feel good about herself and her new normal life.

When you can't be with her in person, add a few personal touches now and then that go beyond routine phone calls. Write her a letter or send her a little present or flowers. If you are more tech savvy, arrange a regular video chat on the computer, or fire off a quick text. The best thing that she can have in her life is a dad who is there for her, by her side, to love her and accept her for the wonderful person she's become after cancer.

. . . .

The New Sister and Brother Life

. . . .

As has been stated throughout this book, sisters often look to their brothers for comic relief, as well as valuable aides to help them handle parents when they get to be too much for her. Breast cancer has put a new wrinkle on the sister–brother relationship. Even though breast cancer statistics are very good—so good that many doctors like to refer to it as "curable"—cancer is still serious business and there are no guarantees. Death, even the threat of it, is scary to everyone, but is especially ominous when it's your own sister who is facing it.

Relating

On first blush, it would seem that a brother is the last person to relate to his sister's breast cancer. Since 99 percent of men never contract the disease, how can he possibly know what she's just been through? Well, the "relating" has to do with the simple fact that they are related—closer, in fact, than anyone else in the family. They grew up together, so who they are, and who they became as adults, has an awful lot to do with their being together as siblings. Your sister may or may not be close to you in age, but you usually have both, or at least one, of the same parents. How you see the big picture was formulated in childhood, together, in the same household.

If you were helping her through treatment, you have a pretty good understanding of what she has gone through to beat cancer. Moving forward, it will be helpful for her to have you in her corner when she faces her fears of cancer coming back, as well. If you weren't around during her treatment, that doesn't mean you can't make it up to her now. Any support that you can give her at this time will be much appreciated.

What if there has been a strained relationship between you two? Ask her forgiveness, and begin to show her how much you care for her and what you are willing to do for her. Being present in her life is the best healing you can offer. Listen to her, and show her your love, which will begin to break down any emotional walls between you.

Relieving

A brother can be so helpful in relieving the daily stresses of her life. So much has been thrown at her, and she needs to lighten up. The transition to "normal life" can be extremely difficult, so you can be there to help. You are in a unique place in her life: you never had responsibility for raising her, nor do you have any romantic responsibilities. In essence, you fall between the cracks of responsibility, so you can be the crack-up, if you will, and bring her joy, mindless behavior, and good old fun.

Refreshing

You need to be her positive light, her beacon of hope, the brother who believes all is well in the new normal life. You are the breath of fresh air that she needs to feel on a regular basis. Send her silly notes, gifts, or jokes; call her on the phone to help her realize that life can be, and should be, about enjoying life.

The New Mom and Son Life

Women are notorious for thinking of others before themselves. This is especially true when it comes to their children. Her kids are the first thing that she thinks about when she lifts her head up from her pillow in the morning and often the last thing she's thinking about when she lays her head down at night. For almost every woman living and breathing today who has children, the title "Mom" is the greatest honor ever bestowed on someone. With that said, over the last few months, at least, breast cancer has taken away her ability to be a full-time caregiver, and that has really frustrated her. She's *so ready* to get past people's feeling sorry for her, their taking care of her, and their worrying about her. She wants to be herself again, and the best way you can help her do that is to be respectful to her as your mom.

Respecting

What does it mean to be a good son? For me, it meant never, ever forgetting that mom is Mom, with a capital M, meaning that there is no person I should respect more (other than Dad, yes big D). Your mom worked so hard to raise you, the least thing you can do for her is to listen to what she wants and needs from you. That doesn't mean you need to do everything that she says you should do. If you did that, you would have never become an adult.

No, what this means is that you have to really listen to what she says, and respect her opinion—whether you agree or disagree with it. Just because you don't always see eye to eye with your mom doesn't mean that you have the right, at this delicate moment anyway, to challenge her, fault her, or worst of all, belittle her. She is, and will always be, your mother. The greatest respect that you can give her is to stay in constant touch and to remember all the important dates in her life.

Remembering

Remember her birthday. Remember Mother's day. Remember Valentine's Day. Remember her wedding anniversary. But most important, remember the day she was diagnosed with breast cancer, which goes a long way to making her feel loved and cared for by you. She is going to worry that it will return, and you need to remind her, on a regular basis, that she is going to be fine; and if for some reason she isn't, you are always going to be there for her. She needs to know that you are her protector as her son, as her shining light.

Responding

It comes as no surprise that moms usually are the initiators of conversations with their sons. They almost always are the first ones to call, the first to write the birthday and holiday notes, the first to visit. That's what they do. They're moms. But as a son, you need to respond, each time she reaches out to you, by returning her calls quickly or responding to her e-mails as soon as you receive them. She is vulnerable right now, so the quicker you can respond when she reaches out to you, the better.

....

The New Friendship Life

....

Nothing puts a friendship under greater pressure than when one friend gets sick. The dynamic in that friendship changes dramatically, with one friend taking the caregiver role and the other the patient role. This can be disruptive to a friendship because, in most cases, friends are on an equal footing—two individuals who trade their care for one another in a seamless and transparent manner. Well, after treatment, your friend is no longer "sick," and so it's time to get your friendship back on an equal footing.

Recovering

With so much pressure on her, and you, there has to be a period of recovery from all that craziness of the cancer process. Perhaps the best thing you can do is to take a little break from each other to get your footing back as friends. You have probably spent a lot of time away from other friends and your family, so tell her that you need a little time away in the coming weeks, now that her cancer treatment is over. She has a lot to process as well regarding how she will move forward, and the best way for her to deal with that is to have some time to herself. That said, if she calls on you, of course you are going to be there for her. But reassure her that she is no longer in Code Red, DEFCON 1 mode. She needs to begin to accept the fact that the war is over, and that both of you need time to replenish your energy.

Relaxing

When you are spending time with your friend now, focus on activities that aren't cancer related. Life, for both of you, has begun anew, so reconnect to what originally drew you together. Go out to your favorite bar together, or cook a meal together, or watch a movie that makes you both laugh. Enjoy the little things that you share.

Reconnecting

Your friendship is now all about spending quality time together, without an agenda or purpose. It's about just being friends again. When you are with her in public, avoid talking about her cancer past. Focus on what she is doing now that cancer is no longer in her world. When she starts to get depressed, help her back up by showering her with optimism and positive energy.

· · · · · · · · · · · · · · · ·

The New Coworker Life

· · · · · · · · · · · · · · · ·

Having just watched a coworker go through her ordeal with breast cancer is a reminder to you (and your fellow coworkers) of your own personal vulnerability to disease—and even more scary, your own mortality. Nobody likes to think about sickness and death, especially at work. Now that she has come back to work full-time, there may be some adjustment time for her, and you, to settle in to the new reality that she is a breast cancer survivor. During this transition period, it may feel a bit uncomfortable, for her and for you, so let those feelings play themselves out naturally, and not forcefully. The most important thing you can do for her is to make her feel welcomed back, fully welcomed back, into her coworker fold, by including her in any and all meetings and events that she would normally be part of. It's time for her, and you, to get back to work as seamlessly as possible.

Recognizing

It's important to recognize the effort she has made during her ordeal by trying to be at work and remain a team player, despite the obstacles presented by her treatment. Acknowledging the contributions that she has made, and continues to make at work, will help her feel more comfortable in getting back to the regular routine at work. She should feel normalcy from her coworkers and bosses, and that she never really left the routine.

Reaffirming

If you are her boss or coworker, this time is for making her feel like the rest of the gang. She is not a special case and was not when she was going through cancer, and will not be in the future as a survivor. She has been, and will continue to be, treated just like the rest of her coworkers. The worst thing that you can do for her is to make her somehow believe she is different because she has had breast cancer.

Returning

Now that the breast cancer regimen is behind her, you should put it behind you, as well. What happened doesn't have to be forgotten, or never talked about, but it should drift into the background. There are more pressing issues—sales, billing, manufacturing, servicing, etc.—all the routine things that happen on your and her jobs. The focus now is on making the mundane special again, to help her get to an acceptance, inside herself, that she truly is cancer free.

CHAPTER 7

The Great Unknown

Will It Return?

．．．．．．．．．．．．．．．．．．．．．．．．．

IT'S OVER. Or is it? For the next five years, at least, it's never fully over. The good news is that as each diagnosis anniversary passes, the cancer drifts further and further into the past. With the treatments now long over, the only thing left for her to do is have her regular checkups and, if she is on hormonal therapy, take a pill or two every day. She's been awarded a full cancer discharge. But for the next five years, she is still going to wonder—is it coming back? Welcome to Cancer Purgatory.

．．．．．．．．．．．．．．

Cancer Purgatory

．．．．．．．．．．．．．．

This is a place that is no place. It has no beginning, middle, or end. It never starts, and never stops. It just is. It is the land of what-ifs. When I was growing up, the Catholic nuns at St. Margaret Mary Elementary School taught me that purgatory was a place where sinners went who weren't all that bad to go straight to hell, but not good enough to get a golden ticket through the pearly gates. It was right smack in the middle of heaven and hell, a way station where petty sinners dwelled until the end of the world for clearance to get into heaven.

Sister Patricia taught me in the third grade that purgatory was white—not a pure white, but a creamy white, thanks to that black bit of sin blended in. Purgatory was the place where its inhabitants went to get purified. Here, the residents had a little pain and suffering, but nothing too bad. The suffering was all about what might happen if God changed his mind about them. So the odds were, in the end, that all would be good, but it wasn't a shoo-in. No doubt, the worst part about purgatory is the wait. It isn't eternity, mind you, but it could be a really long time before the world ends. Thankfully, Cancer Purgatory is not that long. It's only five years, but it sure seems like an eternity. And so your loved one and you wait.

"Nobody ever says that it's (officially) over with breast cancer," according to Jill Taylor-Brown, director of Patient and Family Support Services, CancerCare, Manitoba, Canada. "They say things are good, and unless you have symptoms, you will be fine." The problem is that in Cancer Purgatory, your loved one doesn't feel fine because, according to Taylor-Brown, she always is going to worry whether she is being checked properly.

Psycho-oncologist Dr. Jimmie Holland, in her book *The Human Side of Cancer*, concurs: "We expected women to be jubilant on finishing treatment; in fact, the opposite occurred. They had a paradoxical increase in distress just after treatment, and we learned then about this feeling of vulnerability on finishing treatment. Two main factors caused this new and unexpected anxiety: the fear that the cancer could come back now that they were without the protective effects of treatment, and the fear that they were not being watched as closely by their doctors."

No matter how many mammograms, CAT, MRI, and PET scans she has, no matter how many blood tests, no matter how many genetic tests done, there is no absolute guarantee for her, or you, that the cancer is gone. What the heck can you do, then? Throw a gratitude party.

The Gratitude Party

This is a party not about her, or about you, but about all those who were there for both of you, through thick and thin, during your fight in Cancer Land, and who now need to be recognized for their incredible contributions. The first Gratitude Party I held, with my wife, was on New Year's Day 2002—almost one year to the day after Sharon's breast cancer diagnosis. It was Sharon's idea to bring together our closest friends and family members to celebrate all that they had done. She and I cooked all the food, and bought everyone a leather-bound Journal of Gratitude, a blank book in which we each wrote a comment about how we were grateful to that person for his or her help throughout Sharon's breast cancer treatment.

"I wanted to start the year off right, by paying tribute to all the people who had been key members of our team," according to Sharon. "I wrote a long thank-you for everything I could think of that they did for me. That day, we all sat down in the living room, and I went around the room and thanked each person in detail for what I felt they gave me that was unique to them. It was very emotional—a lot of crying. I remember my friend Jennie putting wads of tissue between her eyeglass frames and her cheeks to catch the tears. I felt great afterwards, and I think everyone else did, too. I also remember Anthony (a firefighter who worked at the World Trade Center site after 9/11), raising his glass and saying that his idea of 'hero' had been redefined by me for him, and that meant a lot to me because he is not very emotional."

The Great Unknown

When all the final cancer checkup appointments have been made, and all the thank-you notes to her and your friends and family have been written, what then? You and she do know a few things. You know from the last chapter, for example, that she is now living in a different world, what I've referred to as the "new normal life." She may be taking hormonal therapy to keep cancer at bay, and she may not. She will get regular checkups and wait, then wait some more. She will have pains that appear. She will worry that they are cancer, and won't really know until she is checked out by her doctors. She will get back to her life, and then wait some more.

All outward evidence says that her cancer is gone. She will look just like every other woman walking down a busy street. No one will know that you had someone close to you go through cancer, either. To the world at large, nothing ever happened. But you know, and she knows, something *did* happen, something so profound that it changed your lives, forever. Now it's time for both of you to look at life and how you're going to live it going forward.

Two years to the day after my wife was diagnosed, we decided to make a huge change in our lives: we moved from the New York City metropolitan area to Roanoke, Virginia, a small city nestled in the Blue Ridge Mountains. Our two boys, Seth and Isaac, were nine and seven at the time, so we decided that, if we were going to make a move, it had to be then. But for us, the adjustment was extreme. To go from the largest and most vibrant city in America to a place of less than 100,000 is drastic, to say the least. But we needed a big change, and we got it.

It took us about eighteen months to make the full adjustment. We continued (and still do) to keep an office in New York City, but our family is now based in Virginia. The move was the right one for us. We were now closer to Sharon's dad and his wife, who adore our kids. And we were able to establish a whole new life with friends who knew nothing about what we went through in Cancer Land.

We take more trips throughout the South, which we love to do. We also traveled much more abroad than we did before, thanks to a lower cost of living, taking the kids to faraway places like Costa Rica, Argentina, France, England, and Italy. Most folks don't make such drastic changes in their lives, and that is fine, too. My sister's big change was moving into a new house down the street. My mom went back to work, as did my mom's best friend, Caryl, after they were finished with treatment.

Life moves on, but the residual fear of cancer returning doesn't. Your loved one is going to wonder if any of the foods she eats, the water she drinks, even the surfaces that she touches might somehow trigger cancer. When she has a headache, is that brain cancer? Sharon, for example, had a headache that lasted a few days. Most people, without cancer, would call this a migraine. She called it a high-alert cancer warning; and so within a week, she was being rolled into the circular tube of an MRI machine for a brain scan. What did they find? Nothing. Was it worth the trip? Absolutely. That's because you never really know until you know. Get used to this—for the next five years, or more. It may at times seem a bit like crying "wolf," but wouldn't you like to have the doctors ready to do battle if it really is a wolf?

. . . .

This Is Not a Drill

. . . .

On the other side of the fence are those loved ones who don't want to know if, God forbid, they actually do have a recurrence of cancer. Their fear of cancer is so overpowering that they refuse regular checkups and periodic tests. This is a bad idea, and something that you need to discourage if your loved one leans in this direction. If she isn't scanned, if she doesn't get her blood work, then the doctors can't know her cancer status. That gives cancer the upper hand in the battle. Cancer is a treatable disease *provided* it is caught early, and treated properly. If, however, it is left to its own devices, without medical intervention, it is going to take over your loved one's body and kill her.

When I was a sophomore in college I had a friend, Dave, who was diagnosed with cancer in his lymph nodes. Dave was one of my best friends in high school; our gang used to hang out at his house while we blasted Aerosmith, Yes, and Beach Boys records (hey, we had eclectic tastes), while we lifted weights in his garage. Dave looked like Charles Atlas; he really did. (If you don't know what Charles Atlas looked like, go to www.charlesatlas.com.) Dave was the epitome of health and fitness—until he got cancer, when he lost his hair, lost all his strength, and was sick, really sick, for six months because of the toxic drugs he was given to keep him alive.

Well, Dave made it through his treatment and went back to school to study computer science when computer science wasn't cool. Dave was one of the smartest people I had ever met. He got his Ph.D. in computer science from the University of Texas, where he was writing software for computers to convert handwriting into type. He was then hired by McKinsey & Company, considered by many to be the best management consulting firm in the world, to become one of their highest rated consultants. Dave was king of the world. He married a beautiful woman from Holland, and was ready to start the perfect family. All things were going great for Dave; nothing could hold him back from becoming one of the most successful technology businessmen ever.

But there was one thing that Dave purposely ignored as his success rocket soared into the business stratosphere: he refused to get tested for cancer. He stopped getting medical checkups. He didn't want to know. He thought that if his health was good, then the cancer was simply not there. Well, Dave was wrong—and it cost him his life, at the tender age of thirty-six. When Dave found out that his cancer had returned, it was too late. The cancer had metastasized to everywhere in his body. He tried everything known to the medical community at that time to stay alive. Thanks to his McKinsey connections, he had doctors as far away as Japan working on his case. In the end, however, there was nothing that they could do for him.

I had been after Dave for a long time to get his cancer checkups. Every time I saw him, I asked him about it. Well, Dave got tired of me asking, so he dropped me as a friend. After two years of not speaking, I realized that friendship meant more to me than a disagreement over how Dave handled his medical responsibilities. So I called McKinsey, asked for Dave, and there was a long pause. "Dave no longer works here," the operator said. I thought that was great news, because I knew that Dave wanted to go out on his own, and one day would start his own tech business with our high school buddy Tommy. So, I asked the operator for Dave's new number. Again, a long pause, this one much longer than the first: "Dave died."

Right before Dave's funeral, his wife had asked that a mutual friend call me to tell me that Dave had passed away, and to inform me where and when the funeral was going to be held. The friend, in his grief, forgot to make the call. Now, two years later, I was finding out about his death from a telephone receptionist. I still haven't been to Dave's grave, so for me Dave's death is without closure—and maybe that's a good thing. It confirmed how important it is for friends and family to continually push their loved ones to get checkups if they have had cancer. I quit pushing when I shouldn't have. I will never *ever* do that again.

. . . .

Handling a Recurrence

. . . .

She's never ready for the news. It comes like a bolt from the sky. She has cancer, again. She is probably alone with her doctor when she's told. After all, it wasn't supposed to come back. But it did. She has been unexpectedly thrown back into Cancer Land.

Why? She was doing everything that she was told to do by her doctors. She was getting her regular checkups, was on her daily drugs, was doing it all right—and now this. Why, why, why? That question again, with the impossible answer.

It's time to go back into battle mode again. The fight is back on to save her life. Before anything else, a determination needs to be made about the cancer itself. Is it localized or has it spread? What protocol do her doctors propose in fighting this next round? Who needs to be told, and when? All the past plans, used in the first round, apply again, with one major difference. With a recurrence, cancer has moved into a new category. It is no longer a curable disease. It has advanced to a higher level. Cancer has become a chronic disease that she must now face for the rest of her life.

That's really heavy stuff to process, and a lot has to be decided over the next few weeks, months, and years. But here's the good news: just because cancer is chronic, it doesn't mean it is a death sentence. That's right. She can live for years, even decades, after a recurrence. Recurrent breast cancer, thanks to the incredible advances seen in medicine over the last three to five years, has been downgraded, in most cases, from a terminal to a chronic condition. Leukemia, diabetes, asthma, epilepsy, multiple sclerosis—all are chronic diseases.

With this said, she has suffered another major shock to her physical and emotional systems. Being diagnosed with cancer is always a big deal, but it's a much bigger deal when it happens again. She is going to need some time to regroup, so give her as much room as possible—in terms of time off from responsibilities, work, kids, and so on. It's time to rally her Cancer Armed Forces. First up, The Corps, to get her ready for her next battle. Right behind them is her Medical Army. She already has the doctors from her original team, and they of course should be consulted. But she needs to give consideration to new members on the medical team. Entering Cancer Land a second time raises the stakes considerably, so she wants to make sure that only the very best Medical Army is available to her.

If she was treated at a local hospital the first time, this is the time to consider physicians and hospitals accredited at Comprehensive Cancer Centers or university medical institutions. Again, her decision on her treatment is final, but the treatment this time has to be spot-on, for the room for error has shrunk considerably. This time, the treatment has to be right. She may not get the opportunity for a third round. Given her prognosis, this also may be the time to seriously consider a clinical trial. Because the cancer has recurred, she can assume a bit more risk in treatment, in the hope that her reward will be stopping the cancer for good.

A recurrence doesn't mean that her life must stop. She can continue her daily life between the treatments. Elizabeth Edwards, wife of John Edwards, demonstrated this better than anyone else. She was in the middle of a presidential campaign with her husband, John Edwards, when it was discovered that she had metastatic breast cancer in her rib, lung, and hip. She continued on the campaign trail between doctor visits and chemo sessions, while her husband pursued his quest for the presidency.

The couple received a lot of criticism for this decision, in no small part because her chances of fighting the cancer were unknown, and they had two small children at home. This, of course, put into question the couple's priorities, with critics saying that they had placed politics ahead of family. Then things really got out of hand for the Edwardses when it was revealed that John Edwards was having an affair with a videographer who was covering his campaign. Psychologists interviewed on various cable news shows speculated that it was Elizabeth's illness that triggered his infidelity, that his fear of losing his wife was strong enough to cause him to act out as a way of distancing himself from her. Whatever the reason, clearly it was the worst thing that he could have done for his wife, given her serious health condition, and it was a selfish act on his behalf. Despite all this, Elizabeth made the decision to remain in her marriage, if for no other reason than to not disrupt her children's lives any more than they already had been.

If your loved one has a recurrence, the treatment might include surgery to remove the tumor or tumors, as well as chemo and radiation therapies, all of this depending on the type of tumor found and its location. When my mom had her recurrence, she was placed on an extremely aggressive chemo regimen, given drugs every week. This made her even sicker than the first time she was treated. Why go through this? She told me that the reason she got out of bed each day was for her family. She still had young children at home, and so she was going to fight until the very end. My mom's best friend, Caryl, also had a recurrence, and also had to face extreme pain and suffering through her treatments, and yet again fought the good fight for her children as well.

The best thing that you can do when she has a recurrence is to give her the hope that she is going to beat cancer, again. This isn't easy to do, especially when you see how sick your loved one is after receiving very aggressive chemo, radiation, and surgical treatments. In more extreme situations, a stem cell transplant may be recommended to save her life. Whatever the medical regimen is, you need to convince her that the fight is worth all the hurt she's feeling. You have to show that she has a lot to live for, and that this will end, just like the first time.

As far as the other members of her Corps are concerned, be sure that they are as positive and upbeat as you are. There will be friends and family who will not project the positive energy she needs, and so they need to be culled from her team. When my mom was going through her recurrence battle, she desperately wanted her parents by her side, especially her mom. But my Nana couldn't face the possibility of losing her daughter, after the loss of her oldest son, Jack, in a tragic drowning accident at the tender age of twenty-one. So Nana just shut my mom out. But Mom was a force of nature, and she never accepted no as an answer. After a major chemo treatment, she got in her car and made a seven-hour drive to talk with Nana, to beg her to be there for her. Along the way, my mom had to pull over repeatedly to vomit because she was so sick from the chemo.

Pressing to finish the drive before dark, Mom ignored the gas tank indicator, and so the car ran out of gas twenty miles from town. She had to walk to a house off the road to call Nana to come pick her up. Nana said that she couldn't come out to get her because she couldn't leave my grandfather, who had a cold. My mom was crushed by this. In that moment, she learned, harshly, that her mom was not part of her Corps, that she couldn't ever be, in no small part because she never resolved the death of her son. My mom never got over the pain that Nana inflected on her. It cut too deep.

Having to face cancer head-on, again, when her mom turned her away at her greatest moment of need, broke my mom's heart. Despite this major setback, my mom was one of the strongest women I have ever known. She adjusted by turning to her best friend, Caryl, also a breast cancer survivor, and to her kids and my dad. Being the oldest of seven in our family, I felt that it was my duty to be there for Mom. So I visited her every chance that I got, which averaged two or three times a month, by catching the Amtrak from Penn Station in New York City to Wilmington Delaware where she lived. She just needed my company while she folded the laundry, or took a walk, or watched her favorite late-night show.

But Mom was losing her battle. The tumors had spread to her pelvis and right breast, and had reappeared again where she had her first mastectomy, this time on her chest wall and in her skin. The tumors were pumping fluid throughout her body, causing her to gain a lot of weight, putting tremendous pressure on the cardial walls of her heart. She was admitted to the hospital in late November, right after Thanksgiving. Tubes attached to her body were dispensing what appeared to be quarts of pale yellow fluid. The cardiologist asked to have a conference with my dad, who asked me to come along with him. "I give her forty-eight hours tops, until her heart gives out," the cardiologist said. "The pressure is too great, and the fluid can't be contained. I would advise that you get things in order as soon as you can."

Get things in order? I don't think the guy could have been more heartless to my dad—and this from a doctor who specializes in treating hearts. My mom already knew what the cardiologist had told us, so when I went back in the room, she grabbed my arm and pulled me close to her. She stared straight past my eyes into my soul (as only moms have the power to do). "What do you think?" she said to me. "Do you think that I am going to die?"

I was speechless. So I just stared right back at her, tears in my eyes.

"I'm not ready to die," she said.

It was then that I realized that what she needed from me was belief—belief that she was going to make it through this impossible medical hell.

"If you don't want to die, then you won't die," I said.

My mom smiled at me and hugged me tighter than I ever remember, despite her weakened state. "Then I won't," she nodded, pulled herself up on her pillow, and kissed me. "I'll show them."

The next day, the cardiologist came into Mom's room while she was sleeping to check her fluid-collection bag. There was nothing in the bag. He reached over to touch her, thinking that she was dead. She jumped up. My mom didn't like to be touched by strangers when she was sleeping, so he was as startled as she was. But that was nothing compared to the surprise he had when he checked my mom's heart. It was beating normally. As for the fluid, it was gone—no trace of it anywhere. The cardiologist had no medical explanation as to how this happened. But Mom did. Her patron saint, St. John Neumann, had come through for her in spades, again. Two days later, Mom checked out of the hospital.

Mom had been making regular visits to the shrine of her self-appointed cancer patron saint, St. John Neumann, ever since she was first diagnosed. When my mom was told that her cancer had recurred, she, my sister Mary, and Caryl, went to see her saint, where his body is encased in glass under an altar, dressed in his finest bishop vestments. My mom, in pain and having difficulty walking, hobbled up to the altar and looked down on the saint, and started praying. Caryl, meanwhile, started threatening: "If you like where you are laying now, you better take really good care of my friend, or else I am going to torch this place of yours," she said. Threatening a saint to help your friend fight cancer—that had to be a first in the cancer-caregiving playbook. But it worked. Mom got better, and Neumann didn't have to face the wrath of Caryl.

That Christmas, which proved to be my mom's last, was a special one, indeed. I didn't have much money at the time, as I was working as a freelance journalist, but I scratched together my savings to buy Mom something that she had always wanted: an emerald ring. I cried as I watched the pure joy that spread across my mom's face when she opened that box, and slid the ring over her finger, turning it back and forth under a nearby table lamp to marvel at the green luminance changing colors with the changing light reflections. Mom, not a Julia Child in the kitchen, cooked the best meal of her life that day: prime rib, mashed potatoes, green beans, and apple pie.

For the moment, my mom's cancer had been beaten—but only temporarily. She continued to believe that she was going to win the battle. It was great that she had such an optimistic outlook, but in that optimism, she had refused to prepare for the possibility that cancer *could* win the war, in the end. After the holidays, I asked my dad about what they had done in terms of their wills—just in case cancer did prevail. My dad looked back at me blankly, and said that Mom didn't have a will, and neither did he.

. . . .

Necessary Preparations

. . . .

Denial, I would argue, is the strongest defense mechanism in human behavior. It's not uncommon, at all, for cancer patients to believe that everything is going to be all right, even in the face of overwhelming evidence that they are going to die. Pam, in her late forties, had first been diagnosed with Stage I cancer, having one lump, and she underwent a mastectomy and chemo for treatment. In her follow-up exams, she was deemed cancer free. Four years later, during a routine exam, large tumors were discovered in her liver, and she was declared by her doctors to be Stage IV.

Pam was married to Frank, and they had three boys. Believing it best not to tell her children, so as not to worry them, she and Frank kept the severity of her condition to themselves. Over the next two years, Pam was placed on an extreme chemo regimen. The treatment seemed to be working; the tumors shrank. Frank threw a big party for Pam's fiftieth birthday. But then, in early December, after an examination, her prognosis got worse: the cancer had spread to her brain. That same day, Frank learned that he had received a huge promotion, to managing director of his company.

Over the next few months, Frank felt that he needed to keep his "eyes on the ball" about two things that seemed directly to conflict with each other: his job and his wife. According to Frank, "I felt like, 'I can't lose my job because I'm not paying attention.' It's a very male thing. I've got to make sure that I'm taking care of the bacon." The rest of the time, "I was trying to take care of Pam, and I think the kids kind of came up short."

Frank's oldest son, Michael, had just turned thirteen and was an "early adopter" of teenage bad behavior. Pam, who because of her serious condition had to treat the cancer "like a full-time job," wasn't able to pay close attention to what Michael and the rest of her kids were up to. Frank, completely focused on his job and his wife, didn't, either. "Michael was drinking, smoking, and lying about it all in a very teenage way." Michael's grades at school plummeted, and he became "unmotivated and 'untogether,'" as Frank recalls.

Meanwhile, Pam's brain meds weren't working, and the cancer kept growing. She was given radiation treatments to her brain. Despite her grim future, Pam refused to tell her kids that she was dying. "Pam was dropping our second son, Jay, off somewhere, and Jay asked, 'Mom, are you going to die?' And she said, 'Nah, don't worry about it.'" Jay was crying out for a discussion about what was going to happen, and Pam was basically blowing him off.

Pam's way of coping with her metastatic cancer was to focus only on the positive. When she would talk with her doctors about her future, she wanted to hear only about patients who were still alive five years later after taking the same brain meds she was taking, and not about the patients for whom it wasn't working, and not the vast majority who had died. "She didn't want to hear the dark side," Frank says. "She told her doctors to only tell her about the good stories. That kept her kind of positive, with an upbeat attitude. But the price of that was that she couldn't go to 'I'm dying and I'm going to die.' And who could blame her for that? Yet the cost was that we didn't do enough to prepare the kids. I knew that she was not going to live forever. The kids didn't know, not at all."

So why didn't Frank just tell the kids himself? "In the last month [of Pam's life], I was out with the guys, at a Subway, and I wanted to say to the kids, 'Guys, mom's dying,' but I couldn't do it," Frank said. "If I did, it would have been a betrayal to her. I should have said, 'Pam, you need to tell the kids.' I kind of deferred to her and I think that was a mistake. But Pam couldn't go there because it would have shattered the way she was dealing with things."

By late May, there was nothing more her doctors could do to save her and she was recommended for hospice care. "All the good options were gone, and she was miserable," Frank remembers. "You keep trying to come up with the space between the side effect and the benefit, and that space is survival. But at some point that space gets to be so narrow that it becomes nonexistent and you can't win."

With the kids still not knowing that Pam's death was imminent, Frank finally decided he had no choice but to tell them himself. "I remember the night I said to Michael that Mom's dying. I finally said it. You can't imagine how hard it was to get it out of my mouth. And he fell apart immediately. 'Why didn't you tell me?' He was crying in bed with Pam, but she was loopy by this point. She was fading in and out." Michael, meanwhile, felt "a sense of betrayal." Two days later, Pam died.

Frank soon realized that he and his wife had made a huge mistake in hiding Pam's inevitable death from their children. "Pam and I used to talk, and she would say 'Frank, what am I going to tell the kids? Hey, I'm going to die soon? What's the point of alarming them? We can't do anything about it.' I see now [that] what to do about it was for us to have told them. They needed time to wallow in their feelings and Pam would be able to say, 'Oh, baby I know it is going to be okay.' All that emoting would have helped them be more healthy emotionally as people. We missed a couple of steps."

Soon after Pam's death, Frank began to date his wife's best friend, Barbara, who had been helping Pam get to doctors' appointments and around the house. Sixteen months later, Frank and Barbara were married. They sold their houses and "merged" their families into a new house. Frank is happily married, but as far as his boys are concerned, "I don't think they are doing very well. The wounds are very real." His oldest son is graduating high school, but his grades are so bad that Frank decided to hold him back from college for a year. Michael continues to suffer from drinking problems, and "his interaction with everybody isn't wonderful." Jay, meanwhile, is suffering from an eating disorder. "He wasn't eating," according to Frank. "He would sit around and have two pieces of bread for dinner," and then later tap into his "private stash of Pop-Tarts in his room with a bowl of ice cream and whip cream at ten o'clock at night." The end result was that "he had fallen off the growth chart." At age 15, Jay was 5'4" and 115 pounds. Frank's youngest son seemed to be doing all right, but he, like his brothers, was "undersocialized." The reasons for all these troubles at home for Frank is pretty straightforward: "I don't think there was the right amount of closure for my sons."

. . . .

The Last Good-Bye

. . . .

Three months after my mom had beaten back cancer, it came back at her with a vengeance. The fluid was back again, putting enormous strain on her heart and kidneys. She was always out of breath, having to stop and rest after a few steps. You could see in her eyes the constant push to find energy inside her body. Her skin was ashen white. The tumors throughout her body hurt her so badly that she could barely walk, or even sit up in the bed; and so the doctors had to heavily sedate her for the pain.

When she entered the hospital, our entire family, along with Caryl, descended on the waiting room where we lived for seven days and nights, around the clock. Every morning, when Mom woke up, she told me that she could beat "this thing," but by the end of every day, her condition got a little bit worse. By the end of the fifth day, everyone knew that death was near. It was time to say good-bye to Mom, for the last time.

On the last day of my mother's life here on earth, Mom said good-bye, individually, to each of her seven children, her best friend, and her husband. Cancer is a very bad thing, but the one good thing about it, when compared to a heart attack or stroke or car accident, is that it does give you the chance to say good-bye to your loved one in a way that you can live with yourself for the rest of your life.

When I walked into my mom's room for my last good-bye, she did what she always did—held out her arms for a big mommy hug. As she pulled me close to her, I started to convulsively cry, which shook the bed so hard that I could hear the bedsprings rattling underneath us. I told her how much I loved her and that I would never forget her. I told her that she was the best mom any child could ever want. I told her that she was the funniest person I ever knew. She told me that she loved me, that she would look after me from above, and that she was going to miss me. The feeling that I had, through this whole experience, was as if I were five years old again and had to leave my mom for the first time to go to kindergarten. Only this time, this five-year-old knew that when he came back from school, she was not going to be home, ever again.

The heaviest thing weighing on my heart, other than losing my mom to cancer, was knowing that my mom would never meet my future wife or children. She shook her head, and said that I had it all wrong. "I'll be there. Don't you worry. I'll be there when the time is right." I had thought that she had lost her mind and had crossed over to the other side right there and then. What I didn't know is that she had planned for that future day already, in a secret conspiracy with her friend, Caryl.

Five years and five months after that fateful day, I was standing in my backyard, holding my newborn son, Seth, in my arms, alongside my wife of one year, Sharon. We were surrounded by family and friends, there for Seth's naming ceremony in the Unitarian Church. Right after the ceremony, Caryl walked up to Sharon and me, and placed over Seth a scapular of St. Francis de Sales, which is a holy card containing the saint's picture and a holy relic. "This is for Seth, from his Grandma," Caryl said. And just like that, Mom had made her promise happen. She truly was with us that day, and every day since, as the scapular hangs between the rooms of my two boys as a constant reminder to everyone in my family of her presence among us.

My mom's scapular is just one example of what cancer patients can do for loved ones before they pass away to pass along their love to future family members. They can make videotapes for their family and friends, or create memory boxes that contain letters and personal items for their loved ones to open during special occasions, such as weddings and childbirths, as a way to keep their presence alive long after death.

On the last day of Mom's life, as she was drifting in and out of consciousness, she suddenly awoke in fright.

"I'm scared. I need my mommy. I need her—*now!*"

My mom, dying from breast cancer in a Newark, Delaware, hospital room, was calling out for her mom—my Nana—to hold her, one last time, before she faced death, head-on. But Nana wasn't there; she wasn't even close. She was 380 miles away in her house in West Virginia because, according to Nana, "I don't know what to do."

Well, I knew what to do. I left my mom with my five brothers and sister, Dad, Aunt Mimi, and Caryl and headed for a phone.

"Hello." Nana answered the phone—thank God.

"Nana, it's John. Mom is calling out for you. She's not going to make it. You need to talk to her."

"We've already been through this. I can't. I'm sorry."

"She needs to say good-bye to you."

"I can't. I just *can'ttt*."

Then, the phone went dead—total silence on the other end. That silence lasted an eternity, until I heard a slight whimper on the other end of the line, followed by convulsive crying. My Nana was about to lose her second child.

Her first, Jack, was a Notre Dame golden boy: college track star, great student, female favorite, all set to attend Notre Dame Law School in the fall of 1953, destined to practice law alongside my grandfather, Jack Yankiss, a prominent prosecutor in Parkersburg, West Virginia. Then one perfect summer day, while goofing around with his buddies and girlfriend in the cold, muddy deep waters of Lake Washington, he told everyone he was drowning. Jack Jr. was up to his old prankster tricks again. Everyone laughed. He went under and never came back up. Nana found out that her son had died that day with a phone call. Now the horror was happening all over again with her daughter Anne.

"As hard as this is, Nana, you're going to have to talk to Mom."

"You can't make me," she yelled back at me through her tears.

"Yes, I can. It's what Mom wants, and she's getting what she wants, if it's the last thing that I do for her. So if I go back into her room, and you aren't talking to her when I get there, the next time you talk to me will be in person when I show up at your door to bring you here by plane, car . . . whatever's necessary. Good-bye, Nana."

I hung up the phone and began my long walk back to Mom's room. I passed by other cancer patients, all of them dressed in hospital gowns, dragging along their IV drips, some walking by themselves, others with a friend or spouse. Then I saw my mom, on the phone. Her face said it all—she glowed, engulfed in pure joy.

"I love you, Mom. I love you so much. I'm really going to miss you too."

Silence, again. Only this time, the entire world had gone silent. I heard nothing. But I sure could feel something, and it was big, really big, welling up from deep inside me. Tears were blinding my eyes. I needed to get out of that room before my mom saw me.

My mom lived and breathed by the sixth sense. She always said that I couldn't hide anything from her. Well, she couldn't ever know what I had just done, under any circumstances. So I left that room, quicker than I came. As I walked away, the tears got bigger, and heavier. My gut wrenched. I was going to vomit in front of all those cancer patients. I leaned over, and . . . someone grabbed me. I looked up. It was my brother, Steve. He had been following me, all the way. He pulled me up, pulled me into his arms, hugging me—real hard—so that I didn't collapse on the floor.

My mom had her mom, and I had my brother.

My mom died around 4 AM on the morning of March 14, 1997. Around her bed stood my dad, my sister, Caryl, and I. I had never seen a person die until then. Mom was choking, coughing, gasping, hacking, and vomiting all night long, and then she just stopped breathing. I touched my mom's hair and face, feeling the warmth of her body leaving her. There was one final rush of air that came from the deepest recesses of her lungs, and then total silence. Her eyes were open, but her pain was closed, forever. She was finally at peace.

When I turned away from that hospital bed, I never looked back. I didn't want to see my mom when she was placed in the casket. I wanted my final memory of her to be as she was, in life, and not death. During her funeral, we kept the casket closed. Ten priests convocated her funeral, which happened on St. Patrick's Day. You would think a bishop had died. The church was overflowing with people, hundreds strong, to honor my mom. The priest who gave the sermon, Father Michael Angeloni, said that my mom led an exemplary life of dignity, grace, and strength—as a breast cancer survivor who fought the good fight for ten long years. Now her fight was over, and it was now time for her to be with her beloved St. John Neumann, forever more.

....

The Odds Are in Her Favor

....

Even though my mom didn't win her cancer battle, three other very important women in my life have: my wife, my sister, and my mom's best friend. Recently, a very close personal friend has been diagnosed, and I'm sure that she is going to whomp cancer's butt as well. The point is that the vast majority of breast cancer survivors *survive* and go on to live healthy, happy, wonderful lives.

Most of these survivors will tell you that getting cancer was the best thing that ever happened in their lives (with the exception of their spouses or children), that it has given them an understanding of life and of their purpose in life that they never would have had before their diagnoses. Breast cancer survivors know better than anyone else how to appreciate life's little gems, and how to live each day in gratitude, fortitude, and humility. As caregivers, we are truly blessed to have our loved ones teach us, by example, how to be better people through their heroic examples as breast cancer survivors. It's no wonder we want to Stand by Her. Who wouldn't?

CHAPTER 8

The War Is Over

Five Years Later

• •

SHE MADE IT. Five years later, and she is still cancer free. Five years is the traditional milestone in the medical community that says, in plain and simple terms, that she beat breast cancer and is cured. Your loved one has finally arrived at the pink ball, and it's time to celebrate. It's time to do something really big for her.

When Sharon hit her fifth anniversary, we decided to take the whole family to Paris and London. The City of Light, aside from maybe Venice (which we went to as well), is the most romantic place in the world. On a night boat cruise down Paris's Seine river, her face glowed as we passed the Cathedral of Notre Dame, while our kids hooted and howled to the people waving to us as we passed under the bridges. Sharon, given her initial diagnosis, was never quite sure if she was going to make the five-year mark. She had friends who never did. Yet here she was, wrapped in my arms—healthy, happy, and fully healed. I was the most grateful husband in the world.

Five years later, my sister is running after her kids, running out the door to her job as a family practice nurse, and running to keep in shape around her beautiful Scottsdale, Arizona, neighborhood. Twenty years later, Caryl is a proud grandmother of four, who works for an eye doctor outside of Harrisburg, Pennsylvania. To honor these special women, and my mom, I wrote a screenplay called *Four Extraordinary Women,* recounting my experiences with them as they each went through breast cancer. Lifetime Television decided that it would be a perfect movie for their Breast Cancer Awareness Month programming in October, so they introduced me to a television producer, and six months later the film was being shot in Canada.

Lindsay Wagner played my mom. Think about that for a minute. How many guys can say their mom is the Bionic Woman? Most of the storyline was changed from the truth—that's what movies almost always do—but there was one scene that still hits me right in the gut. It's when Sharon is being wheeled down a hospital hallway toward her operation, as I am walking alongside her; she looks up at me, reaches out for my hand, and says, "You aren't going anywhere are you?" I look down at her. "No." Then she's gone, and I'm left to myself, looking in a hospital mirror. Why me?

We know by now what to do with those why questions, right: throw 'em straight into the trash. But sometimes—very rarely—the answer to the whys of life become clear. It came to me right after the first airing of my movie on Lifetime. Because of all of the women in my life who had faced breast cancer, I was meant to help men face their fears, angers, anxieties, griefs, isolations, and sufferings when they faced the breast cancers of their wives, moms, sisters, daughters, friends, and coworkers.

So I started writing this book, and I finished it on the exact date that my wife was first diagnosed eight years before. I'm pretty superstitious about breast cancer dates, and I have good reason to feel that way. Sharon, for example, received her first chemo treatment on March 14, the same day that my mom died. And then there is March 17—St. Patrick's Day—the day of my mom's funeral. Every year, I always felt blue on the greenest day of the year. But this year, on March 17, my associate editor Erika Spelman told me that this book was going to be published in October for Breast Cancer Awareness Month. I couldn't believe it. My mom had done it again. At that moment, after twenty-one years, I was no longer enclosed in a sea of melancholy blue over my mom's death, but instead was suddenly enveloped in a streaming double helix of positive pink and green energies, coming straight from the heart of my loving mother.

The fight against breast cancer continues, and will continue until a cure is found. As diagnostic screenings get better, and as the baby boomers get older, more women will be diagnosed with breast cancer. For me, and you, our job is to be the best caregivers to our loved ones we can. But our work doesn't stop there. We also need to help the millions of men who are now entering Cancer Land with their loved ones, to teach them how to Stand by Her.

Sharon and I turn 50 this year, and the house that we live in turns 100. So we decided that the best thing we could do to celebrate all three of our birthdays was to plan a big birthday bash on Halloween night, the last day of Breast Cancer Awareness Month.

The party's theme is "Dress to the Nines." The idea is that everyone invited to our Halloween bash must dress the way people dressed in their favorite year ending in 9. There was a moment when we thought it wasn't such a good idea to throw a big party during these tough economic times. But then the bigger picture became clear to us. If cancer teaches us anything, it is this—why not now?

The people of Costa Rica have a saying that they've trademarked as their national slogan: *pura vida*—the literal translation being "pure life." But the real meaning of the phrase, according to the Costa Ricans, is that *pura vida* is a command to live life, every day, "full of life." Now that her cancer is no more, get out into that great, big world and live life to its fullest—today, tomorrow, this week, next week, next month, next year, and for the rest of your and her days.

www.standbyher.org   Where men connect when their loved ones have been diagnosed with breast cancer.

www.menagainstbreastcancer.org   Men's support site, "caring about the women they love."

www.cancer.gov   National Cancer Institute—lists Comprehensive Cancer Centers, available clinical trials, and valuable medical data and information for patients and doctors alike.

www.breastcancer.org   Medical and support resources, created by Dr. Marisa Weiss, a radiation oncologist.

www.cancer.org   The official site of the American Cancer Society with valuable information about breast cancer.

www.drsusanloveresearchfoundation.org   Up-to-date breast cancer research, founded by Dr. Susan Love, a breast cancer surgeon and researcher.

www.abms.org   American Board of Medical Specialties, which provides information about physician qualifications and certifications.

www.komen.org   Susan G. Komen for the Cure, a support and advocacy organization committed to finding the cure for breast cancer.

www.healthgrades.com Provides detailed information about physician qualifications, malpractice actions, years of practice, etc.

www.bestdoctors.com Peer reviews of physician qualifications, started by doctors from the Harvard University School of Medicine.

www.adjuvantonline.com Resource for patients with early cancer diagnoses to analyze the risks and benefits of adjuvant therapy—chemotherapy, hormone therapy, or both—after surgery.

www.ibcsupport.org Inflammatory breast cancer help and support.

www.cancercare.org Provides free professional support services for anyone affected by cancer.

www.cancerhopenetwork.org Support for cancer patients and their loved ones that links individuals to other patients/loved ones who have had similar experiences.

www.gildasclub.org Founded in memory of comedian Gilda Radner, this organization provides free social and emotional support to cancer patients, family, and friends, with clubs in cities throughout the United States and Canada.

www.sharecancersupport.org SHARE—survivor-led support for women with breast or ovarian cancer, their families, and their friends.

www.networkofstrength.org Support resource for patients diagnosed with breast cancer.

www.caringbridge.org "Free personalized websites that support and connect loved ones during critical illness, treatment and recovery."

www.thestatus.com A free service that connects patients to their friends and family and provides information about their patient's medical condition.

www.lotsahelpinghands.com Free web-based community that organizes family, friends, neighbors, and colleagues to help a patient and the patient's family when in need.

www.corpangelnetwork.org   Arranges free air transportation for cancer patients traveling for treatment, using empty seats on corporate jets.

www.mamm.com   "Women, Cancer and Community."

www.nccam.nih.gov   National Center for Complementary and Alternative Medicine.

www.youngsurvival.org   "Young Women United Against Breast Cancer."

www.thewellnesscommunity.org   "Cancer Support, Education and Hope," which provides group counseling, educational programs, and exercise, nutrition, and relaxation classes in centers across the United States.

www.livestrong.org   Uniting "people to fight cancer, believing that unity is strength, knowledge is power, and attitude is everything."

www.cisforcupid.com   "Online dating for people affected by cancer."

http://csn.cancer.org   Cancer Survivors Network, provided by the American Cancer Society.

www.lymphnet.org   National Lymphedema Network—support for and about lymphedema.

www.baldisbeautiful.org   Created by survivor Sharon Blynn, this website embraces "bald is beautiful" as a mantra of female self-love and empowerment.

www.fertilehope.org   "Dedicated to providing reproductive information, support and hope to cancer patients and survivors whose medical treatments present the risk of infertility."

www.nhpco.org   National Hospice and Palliative Care Organization providing information about hospice care.

www.lbbc.org   Living Beyond Breast Cancer—helping women with breast cancer learn how to cope with their disease and how to live better lives after diagnosis.

www.cancerandcareers.com   An online resource for working women with cancer.

www.facingourrisk.org   FORCE—for women, and their families, whose family history and genetic status puts them at a high risk for breast and/or ovarian cancer.

John W. Anderson is the president and founder of The Farm, an advertising and production company with offices in New York and Virginia. He is an Emmy-nominated director of television commercials, including Lifetime Television's "Stop Breast Cancer for Life" campaign, and a writer, producer, and director of television shows. He is an attorney licensed to practice in New York and Virginia, specializing in entertainment and business law. He is also a writer for newspapers and magazines whose work has appeared in *The New York Times, Rolling Stone, The Nation*, and many other publications. He has helped his wife, mother, sister, and a close friend in their battles against breast cancer. John is married to Sharon Rapoport and they have two sons—Seth and Isaac—along with a dog named Ginger and three tanks of fish (that remind him, daily, about the need to go scuba diving).

• • •

To learn more about how you can Stand by Her, and to talk with other men about what you are going through privately and anonymously, go to www.standbyher.org.